DEEP SLEEP HYPNOSIS

Hypnosis for Calming Anxiety & Living with Ease

Table of Contents

INTRODUCTION

It is important to have a night's sleep that is good to be able to work and think with a clear head. Remember the soundness of your childhood sleep? Waking up at dawn's crack, feeling completely rested and energized? As we grow, it becomes harder to enjoy the benefits of deep sleep. While some people may associate with anxiety a lack of quality sleep, medical experts agree our growth hormones play a vital role in how well we sleep.

Everyone must rest. Everybody gets a degree of sleep every night, but the value of how much you sleep-and how well-can have a much more significant impact than how awake you feel in the morning. Besides, some interesting associations between deep sleep and type 2 diabetes have been shown in the study. Deep sleep increases the regulation of blood sugar, increases the control of hunger hormones, and increases metabolism. Beautiful stuff, this sleep!

Most people assume that they only have one or two dreams while they sleep at night, and this should only happen when they're in a deep sleep. The reality is that dreaming is far more complicated than you might think, and more than one might imagine, too. Dreaming is a mechanism that assists you with stress and regeneration and is much more important than you think.

But what do the experts consider to be the sleep of a' good' night? Well, how many of us at first light have to drag us out of bed? If you've been sleeping' value,' you will wake up feeling refreshed and ready to go, not more exhausted than before you went to bed the previous night. If this is you, then regularly, you probably won't get enough quality sleep.

CHAPTER ONE

What Do We Understand About Sleep?

Put, Sleep is shutting off the outside world from our experience.

Yet Sleep is complicated as well. Let's look at how we sleep and pass through the different stages of Sleep. The moment the sun goes down, your body starts to prepare for Sleep. The pineal gland begins to secrete more and more melatonin as the light levels decrease. Melatonin is often considered the primary sleep hormone of the body. Melatonin's rising level has a relaxing and soothing effect. Remember when you went camping. You might have been sitting in the dark with thousands of stars overhead in front of a fire. The fire's crackling and heat have an entrancing effect, distracting your mind from your worries. The melatonin's darkness coaxes you to sleep.

Falling Asleep

Once you're in your warm sleeping bag, your mind starts drifting, and you're starting to forget the outside world. You reach Stage 1 sleep now. Slower theta waves replace the stronger alpha waves of the full waking state. Simultaneously, your body becomes more relaxed. Your breathing is starting to slow down, your heartbeat is becoming more steady, and your blood pressure is beginning to fall. The blood flow to your brain begins to decline as well as the temperature of your brain. You can quickly wake up at this stage, and you may even feel you've never really got to sleep.

Light Sleep

You go down to Stage 2 sleep for the next 15 to 20 minutes. If your brain were monitored, a new set of characteristic brain waves would now be shown. Your senses continue to disengage from the external environment, and you wouldn't wake up as quickly at this stage. If someone pushed an eyelid back, you would be unaware of the outside world, seeing nothing. But you may still wake up to a noise in the hall. Most of your body organ systems keep slowing down (low blood pressure, heart rate, muscle tension, secretions of the body).

Deep Sleep

Your brain wave habits change again about 30-45 minutes after sleeping, so for the first time, the deep sleep delta waves emerge. You're now moving into deep sleep stages 3 and 4. (Stage 3 and 4 are separated from each other only by the amount of Beta pulse endeavor measured in the brain. Together they're called deep sleep.) At this stage, it would take a lot of effort to wake you up- only loud noises, and some jostling would wake you up. If at this stage, you are awakened from sleep, you might be groggy, even confused or disoriented, as if you were drunk from Sleep. You may not have been able to work typically for a while. During deep sleep, sleepwalking, talking, or bed-wetting usually occurs. The structures of your body have slowed down to the most profound state of physical rest at this stage of Sleep.

The Deep Sleep Rejuvenating Effects

 While your body replenishes and repairs itself in deep Sleep. The hypothalamus (part of the brain) at this point suggests that the anterior pituitary gland at the base of the brain enhances the release of the human growth hormone (HGH). (HGH is sometimes referred to as the hormonal "youth fountain" due to its ability to restore adult bodies to a more youthful state. Tissues was promotes to building and growth in children.)As your body cycles in and out of deep sleep throughout the rest of the night, additional HGH spurts are released. The overall metabolic activity of the brain diminishes during deep Sleep.

Rapid eye movement sleep (REM)

The brain waves change again after a time of deep Sleep, and the eyes start fluttering back and forth under closed eyelids. You're dreaming now, moving into what's called REM sleep (for Rapid Eye Movement). It has been shown that REM sleep is vital for memory consolidation of recent experiences. There is an increase in blood flow to specific brain areas during REM sleep. These areas include the areas where visual stimuli are processed and the information of our senses. This can explain the vivid nature of the dreams that we often experience. During REM sleep, the blood flow to the prefrontal cortex that governs our ability to assess and analyze experiences remains decreased. This might explain why we embrace the most strange dream material when we're dreaming.

Sleep Cycle

You keep cycle through stages II, III, and IV of unconscious sleep through the rest of the night, then back to dreaming three or four times with Rapid Eye Movement. With each sleep cycle, your brain releases pulses of human growth hormone to regenerate and rebuild my body as you pass into deeper Sleep. This is followed by more dreaming, helping your brain integrate the memory and knowledge of your recent experiences.

Preparing For Daytime Activity

As the dawn light begins to reveal that the morning approaches, your brain stops producing as much melatonin as it does. But how can that be? Your eyes are closed after all. Researchers found that the brain responds to the skin's light. Researchers were able to measure significant changes in the circadian rhythm of the brain as scientists shone a light on the back of the volunteer knee. That's the light that stimulated biological clock changes in our brains.

In the early morning hours before we wake up, numerous other hormonal changes occur. The increase in cortisol is one of the first differences. The brain starts signaling the hypophyseal gland, which in effect, instructs the adrenal glands to release cortisol. Cortisol mobilizes and increases blood sugar in our energy stores. This increased supply of blood sugar is the fuel for our brain, for our internal organs, and for our muscles to get us to wake up.

The Insomnia Stress Connection

We said the brain is signaling the brain with a message to the adrenal glands to wake up in the morning. The cortisol is secreted by the adrenal glands, which raises blood sugar. The adrenal gland is part of the body's response to stress. During stress, the same brain sequence that wakes up in the morning also works (with slight variations on a theme). When your body becomes stressed, cortisol rises. Local hormonal changes also occur within the brain with stress.

The stress response purpose is to prepare you for activity and keep your alertness. The approach to pressure is intended to help us cope with acute crises. When the crisis ends with the stress response, the body de-stresses, and the stress hormone levels return to normal. We often have higher levels of stress hormones all the time with the chronic stresses of modern life.

Because the function of stress hormones is to keep you alert in part, at night, they can also save you alert. That's keeping you awake and keeping you from sleeping. The most common cause of insomnia is stress.

For more information on the connection between stress and insomnia and the importance of our sleep cycles, please visit[

http:/sleepherb.net] Several natural products have been shown to reduce or buffer the stress response in both animals and humans. These are primarily spices, but they also contain vitamins and minerals. Herbs like ginseng, Rhodiola, ashwagandha, licorice root, and others are referred to as adaptogens because they help the body adapt to stress. Adaptogenic herbs are an essential part of any natural strategy for remedying insomnia and encouraging healthy sleep rejuvenation.

Hypnotize to Sleep

Many people have sleeplessness. Perhaps you are curious why hypnosis can help you sleep very quickly.

First, we need to distinguish between everybody knows the "real sleep" and hypnotic sleep, which is also known as "hypnotic trance." Hypnotic traces are a condition between full consciousness and "false sleep." It is a natural state of mind that everybody encounters subconsciously every day.

To attain a deep sleep, we must, first of all, undergo a hypnotic phase. You might wonder at this point how you can go into a deep trance. There are many ways to become hypnosed. All inductions focus your attention on allowing your subconscious mind to obtain information without filters of the conscious mind. You could search for them on Google to find some good self-hypnosis tutorials. I'll post some videos, but this isn't the subject of this chapter

Once you're in a trance, you'll go faster and faster when you don't give any more suggestions. The trance will automatically deepen, and you will fall to the "real sleep" when the trance gets deep.

It takes just a few minutes and is much quicker than waiting for sleep. You can use it anywhere you want to sleep quickly: take a bus, ride or fall asleep at night.

As you're well versed in the idea of self-hypnosis, you can offer yourself suggestions like, "The next time I wake up, I'm going to be refreshed, fully awake."

The Benefits of Sleep Hypnosis

For our lives as human beings, sleep is vital, and indeed it is essential to all living things. We need to sleep well for at least 6 hours to regenerate our bodies and wake up for the next day with renewed energy. It's widespread, however, that we find it hard to sleep soundly. Hypnosis of sleep can help us achieve this.

Hypnosis lets us relax our thoughts. Hypnosis is a therapy that leads to a relaxed state of mind and reaches into our subconsciousness. Most sleeping patients use drugs that have reported side effects, such as grumbling in the night. On the other hand, sleep-induced hypnosis is safe and known to work in the treatment of sleeping disorders.

Everything is about "sleeping like a log" state. Why let your life be ruined by sleep privation if you can do something about it?

Several factors may lead to a disturbed sleep pattern in our increasingly smooth society. There are known factors, such as pressure at work, marital problems, and financial distress. Sleep disturbances lead to inadequate night. Those with sleeping problems usually get exhausted and unable to focus on what lies ahead the next day. If a person doesn't have a quality sleep for 6 or 8 hours, he or she will be slow or exhausted on the following day, which can result in irritability, inability to focus, impatience and poor work results. This could add up to the mounting stress of a person.

Hypnosis is considered to be an excellent way to treat sleeping disorders. This way, a person can relax and regulate the mind to get a good sleep. Hypnosis allows us to touch our subconscious mind and discover the source of our fear and hesitation. This therapy guides our minds to relieve our worries, to relax, and concentrate on this calm state. A person wakes up with good sleep during the night, revitalized and optimistic, prepared for another demanding day.

Sleep hypnosis turns sleeping disorders into a healthy pattern of sleep. This method stimulates our subconscious into a deep state of rest, rest, and sleep, thus keeping a person sufficiently energetic in the morning. We don't have to take drugs such as tablets or drinks to sleep well. We only have to calm our minds and bodies and rejuvenate ourselves with our well-deserved rest. This treatment can help us to sleep like a baby.

Our sleep problem can be reduced by taking part in activities that relax our minds and bodies. Such behaviors differ among individuals. It is also essential that we do not have disturbances such as sound, light, and even televisions at bedtime. We must get rid of the factors that contribute to our sleeping problems. We must finely adjust our body to make it relax.

The most important thing is that we should know why we can't sleep well. We should free our minds from these problems so we can sleep well at night. Sleep hypnosis not only attempts to identify the problem, but it also tries to find a better solution. The most important thing is that we should know why we can't sleep well. We should free our minds from these problems so we can sleep well at night. Sleep hypnosis not only attempts to identify the problem, but it also tries to find a better solution.

Why Sleep Matters - Are You Getting Enough?

If you don't get sufficient sleep (and several millions of us weren't), you have to understand why and what you can do.

You sound as if you never shut your eyes some days. Or you fall asleep, then wake up and watch the clock. If this sounds familiar, you frequently get away from a good night's sleep. This can mean more than just some grogginess for the next day. Too little sleep causes your health, relationships, and work to be thrown and turned and can even jeopardize your safety.

Tossing and turning don't just make you tired of getting enough sleep. It also reduces:* decreases the ability to concentrate* decreases the time of your reaction* increases your memory lapses and your forgetfulness* increase your likelihood of accidents and injuries* increases mood* increasing your susceptibility to sleep BENEFITS OF SLEEP illnesses New evidence shows, for example, that sleep is vital to strengthening your memory and thinking. Sleep also affects mood and plays a pivotal role in healthy endocrine and immune systems in your body that regulate the release of crucial hormones and help protect your body from disease.

Too little sleep is associated with several serious health problems, including hypertension (high blood pressure), obesity, diabetes, heart disease, alcohol consumption, and depression. Being deprived of sleep can also make it difficult to concentrate, make decisions, and create new memories.

Failure to sleep can otherwise damage your health. Drowsy driving is likely to cause more than 100,000 car crashes and more than 1,500 deaths every year reported by police. Poor sleep costs workers in reducing productivity and also increases the risk of injuries at work.

LATE AT NIGHT YES WIDE OPEN?

Several insomnia triggers...

Depression and Stress Anxiety* Use stimulants* Cronymic pain (for the care of the loved person)* Changes in the world* Sleep / Wake cycle interruptions* Medical side effects* Sleep / Wake schedule* Gold, childbirth, and menopause (for women)* Changes in Cycle* Economic noise

While sleeping habits vary wildly, adults are advised to sleep for 7 to 9 hours per night by sleep experts the next day. The' efficiency' of your night, however, always matters. Your sleep must be uninterrupted, not disturbed by repeated awakenings, to renew yourself. You also need sufficient sleep to avoid sleep deep-this is the collective effect of not getting enough sleep over time.

If your sleepiness interferes with your daily activities, you likely need more shut-eye!

STATES AND SLEEP STAGES When you sleep, typically, you go through five stages of sleep: 1, 2, 3, 4, and REM (rapid movement of the eye–also known as' sleeping dreams'). It takes 70-90 minutes for a sleep cycle to pass. You typically have four to six cycles a day. You are almost awake at the end of each cycle before the cycles begin again.

Stage 1: Light sleep, drift into

Stage 2: Help refresh the body

Stage 3: deep sleep entering; Stage 3 and

 Stages 4 are the most restored stages Stage 4: deep sleeping, produces more cells and breaks down proteins; you may feel groggy or disoriented Stage 5 when you are awakened: REM (Dream Sleep) stimulates brain parts used for learning; breathing is faster, irregular, and annoys Relax before sleep. Before bedtime. Train yourself to relax with sleep and make it part of your bedtime ritual. Try a warm bath, a deep breath, pictures, or lectures.

2. Get regular practice. Get daily practice. Exercise every day for 30 (or more) minutes. Until going to bed 3, exercise at least five t six hours — caffeine Clear Steer. Caffeine is an incentive. Don't eat caffeine every day, including coffee, chocolate, soft drinks, teas, prescription medications, and caffeine-containing pain relievers.

4. Make it cozy and dark. Have comfortable soft linens and curtains to block outdoor lights.

5. Alcohol limit. Alcohol can steal you from a deep sleep and keep you in a lighter, less restful period of sleep.

6. Maintain a pleasant room temperature. Too hot or too cold can interrupt your sleep or prevent your sleep.

7. Don't lie there. Don't lie there. The fear of not sleeping may contribute to insomnia. If you can not sleep, get out of bed and do anything else calmly until you are tired.

8. Get up with wind. Wake up with the moon. Sunlight helps to reset the internal clock of your body every day.

9. Set a sleep program. Go to bed every night and get up every morning at the same time.

IDENTIFY A SLEEP PROBLEM While you have occasional sleepless nights, if you are having trouble falling or sleeping at least three days a week, you need to tell your doctor about them. Your sleeplessness can be a form of insomnia, but it can also be a sign of a medical condition or other sleeping disorders.

CHAPTER TWO

Sleep-The Often-Overlooked Tool for Quality Living

Sleep is important for the health and well-being of a person, According to the National Sleep Foundation,.

It's as important to sleep as food and air. To support all growth, human life brain function, and development, it is a necessary function.

Sleep keeps your mind calm and alert. This allows you to work optimally daily.

If you awaken tired after eight hours of sleep or longer, you don't need more sleep. What is needed is a better quality of sleep rather than more rest. Deep sleep is the body's most important type of sleep.

What's sleeping?

Sleep has classified a block of the period when you're not awake for a long time. But sleep studies over the past several decades have found that sleep has distinctive night-wide stages that cycle. Your brain remains active throughout your sleep, but during each stage, different things happen.

For example, the next day, you feel well-rested, and energetic at one stage, and you learn or make memories at another stage.

People usually cycle many times through the different stages during a normal night.

How much sleep is sufficient?

The ought for sleep varies from person to person. Throughout the life cycle, these needs vary.

Every night, most adults require 7-8 hours of sleep.

From 16 to 18 hours a day, newborns sleep. Children are sleeping between 10 and 12 hours a day in the preschool.

However, after as little as six hours of sleep, some individuals can function without sleep or drowsiness. Others, unless they've slept for ten hours, can not perform at their peak.

Some people think that as they get older, adults need less sleep. But there is no proof that older people will sleep less than younger people. It's also easier for older people to wake up.

Research suggests that many people can be convinced that six or seven hours of sleep are all right. Whether you're sleeping or alert throughout the day is the acid test for enough sleep. If you're safe, your sleep is likely to be adequate. But it is more important to sleep than you might think.

Why do you sleep well?

Is it essential if you're getting enough sleep? Yes, yes. Both the quality and quantity of sleep is crucial, but also the quality of your sleep.

In other words, how well you are relaxed and how well you work the next day depends on your sleep time and how much you get each night from the different stages of sleep.

Performance: To think clearly, react quickly, and create memories; we need to sleep. Indeed, when we sleep, the brain pathways that help us learn and remember are very active.

It's a price to skimp on sleep. Cutting back by even 1 hour may make focusing on the next day difficult and may slow down your response time.

Researchers also find that you are more likely to make bad decisions and take more risks when you don't sleep. This can result in lower work or school performance and a higher risk of a car crash.

Mood: Sleep affects mood, as well. Insufficient sleep could make you irritable and is associated with poor behavior and relationship problems, particularly among children and adolescents.

Health: for good health, sleep is also essential. Study show that not getting enough sleep or regularly having poor quality sleep increases the risk of high blood pressure, heart disease, and other medical conditions.

Additionally, the body produces essential hormones during sleep. Deep sleep triggers more growth hormone release, fueling children's growth, and helping to build muscle mass and repair children's and adults ' cells and tissues.

Other type of hormone which increase during sleep work to combat different infections. This may explain why a night's sleep that's good prevents you from getting sick and helps you heal when you get sick.

Sleep's Different Stages consist of various stages.

Stage 1: It is the first ten-minute period of light sleep (drifting away from wakefulness).

Stage 2: It's more profound, and it's 20 minutes long.

Stages 3 and Four: These are forms of deep sleep that come after this.

Stage 4: is the first sleep period. It is also known as non-REM sleep (REM-rapid eye movement). You are "drifting off" in this period.

Stage 1 NREM Sleep is characterized by o Breathing becomes slow, and even o The heartbeat becomes regular

Stage 2: it is an intermediate sleep stage. It's about 20 minutes long. You are gradually going down deeper into sleep, becoming increasingly detached from the outside world.

Stage 2 is characterized by: o Larger brain waves and sometimes rapid activity bursts.

- You're not going to see anything even if your eyes are open.

Stage 3: It's the start of deep sleep. After you fall asleep for the first time, it lasts about thirty to forty-five minutes.

O Brain waves characterize stage 3 are slow (ranging from 0.5 to 4 per second) and relatively large (five times the wave size in Stage 2). These waves of the brain are called delta waves.

O Compared to stage 1 and 2 sleep, you're much harder to wake up. It takes a louder noise to wake you up or an aggressive effort.

Stage 4: During Stage 4, the deepest sleep occurs. It is characterized by o Brain waves (called delta brain waves) that are quite large, giving the EEG a sluggish, jagged pattern.

- Artificial oblivion encounters the sleeper. Those activities will start in this phase if the sleeper is a sleepwalker or a bed wetter.
- Corporal functions continue to decline to the highest level of physical rest possible.
- This is the absolute first cycle of deep sleep. The sleep awakened from deep sleep will likely be tired, disoriented or confused. She or He may experience "sleep inertia" or "sleep drunkenness," which for quite some time, seems unable to function normally.

The sleeper returns to Stage 2 after the first phase of deep sleep is over and then enters the REM state.

REM Sleep Stage Your brain will suddenly become much more active when you enter the REM stage.

REM State Brain wave characteristics are small and irregular, with large eye activity bursts. At this time, the activity of the brain wave is more like waking than it is sleeping.

Progressive relaxation characterizes the four NREM phases. But during the REM phase, the activity of the body is significantly improving.

- Blood pressure may be dramatically increased.
- Pulse rates rise irregularly o Breathing becomes irregular, and the consumption of oxygen increases.
- You can twitch your mouth, toes, and hands.

Usually, the first REM period is brief. The sleeper may wake up shortly after this. It's quite normal. The next day, a good sleeper might not remember it. However, at this point, a poor sleeper may wake up and have trouble getting back to sleep.

It has been shown that Deep Sleep relieves symptoms of insomnia, nervous stress, nausea, anxiety, and depression. To replenish our bodies and minds, deep sleep is essential.

The body heals itself during deep sleep by producing growth hormone that speeds up nutrient and amino acid absorption to help tissue healing.

For physical renovation, hormonal regulation, and growth, deep sleep is crucial. The part of sleep that our brain and body need to recover from the day is a deep sleep. It is sometimes referred to as delta sleep after the brain generates the delta waves.

Deep sleep is our restorative sleep that rejuvenates our bodies from the wear and tear of the day. Deep sleep is much quieter and more relaxing.

Deep sleep is a time of dramatically also reduced blood flow and brain energy use, which is probably crucial to restoring energy which is used in daily self-conscious awareness (e.g., thinking).

Waking up from deep sleep is very difficult because the brain has turned off its external world awareness. The deepest of all the stages is a deep sleep. During this stage, physical regeneration occurs above all.

How to get the rest of a good night?

If you're having trouble sleeping, you're not alone. Field data suggest that it is hard for millions of people to fall asleep.

Simple changes in your daily habits can go a long way to getting better sleep consistently.

During sleep, several vital tasks help maintain good health and enable people to function at their best. Not getting enough sleep can hurt the performance of memory, health, and mood. A good night's sleep is vital to your well-being, like eating well and being physically active. There are techniques for combating common sleep problems, according to leading sleep researchers:

1. Have a regular schedule for sleep/wake
2. Develop a proper bedtime and go to bed every night
3. 3 at the same time. Regular exercises can help you sleep better for about 30 minutes a day.
4. Too much alcohol or caffeine consumption can disturb sleep.
5. Creating a better environment for sleep: no or low noise, low or no light— keep room dark
6. Without strong drafts, let the room be a little cooler and airy. It's not supposed to be stuffy or hot.
7. Even on holidays, observe a regular bedtime schedule.
8. Before you go to bed, eat at least 2 hours. Food digestion may interfere with sleep if you sleep right after eating.
9. Likewise, sleep can be disturbed by too much salty, sweet, fatty food at dinner time.
10. Too many liquids just before going to sleep or 2 hours before going to sleep mean frequent bathroom visits. Too many juices should be avoided.

11. Before you go to bed, relax. Take some time to relax. Before going to bed, have a ritual: read, meditate, listen to music that is soft and soothing.
12. If you still have trouble sleeping, consult a doctor. You should be able to help your family doctor.

The Importance Of Healthy Sleep

Healthy sleep is just as crucial for health as feeding, exercising, and managing stress.

Most Americans fail to make an effort to get healthy sleep, assuming it is costly to sleep. Work is starting to show us this is not true. At our own risk, we are losing sleep.

"There is plenty of persuasive evidence to support the claim that sleep is the most significant indicator of how long you're going to live, maybe more important than smoking, exercising, or having high blood pressure or cholesterol levels."(1) Believe it or not, getting healthy sleep...

Can improve your ability to think clearly and function at the highest level* Can boost athletic performance by 30%* Improves your health and appearance* Helps you lose weight* Improves your memory and learning abilities* Decreases your risk of diabetes* Helps protect your heart and decrease your risk of heart disease* Improves your ability to fight diseases* Decrease your risk of diabetes*

We have always known logically that sleep is essential. "Nothing is safer than the sleep of a good night" is a common expression of this understanding. But we're not listening to our own experience for some reason. Most of us, as children, had a bedtime that was the household law. Our parent made sure we had enough sleep. They knew for us what was right. Most of us appear to have forgotten or ignored the value of sleep as we got older. We live in a culture that respects laboriousness, energy, and efficiency and frowns on lethargy.

There has been a spike in media attention on healthy sleep and insomnia in just the past year (2008). This is mainly due to further research on the ill effects of insomnia on previously unsuspected conditions such as heart disease, diabetes, cancer, obesity, and weight gain. Researchers now suggest that, for these diseases, insomnia is a significant risk factor.

Why do we miss so much sound sleep?

Stress and overwork is a significant cause of lost sleep.

A common reaction in stressful times in our lives is to revive ourselves to meet the demands placed on us. Stresses in our individual lives can come and go. But now it seems that our whole culture is being stressed. Nearly nobody would argue that we are currently experiencing historical relative pressure (around 2008).

Healthy sleep is one of the first stress injuries. We Americans are struggling more than ever with insomnia. A National Sleep Foundation survey found in 2005 that less than half of all

Americans feel they are getting healthy sleep either every night or every other night(5).

The lack of healthy sleep in our nation is reflected in our use of sleep medicines. In 2006, 49 million sleep medicine prescriptions were written(3). This was an improvement of 53 percent over the last five years. The leading sleep drug is Ambien, which in 2006 accounted for 60% of sleep prescriptions or sales of $2.8 billion. Drug companies invested $600,000,000 on ads in 2006. All advertising has focused primarily on "destigmatizing the use of sleeping pills" (5).

While stress is the main reason for all our sleeplessness, our modern surroundings also discourage sleep.

Human-made inventions and artificial light give us many reasons to remain awake at night. Note that the darkness of night put a real damper on staying awake to the wee hours for most of human history.

The inventor of the electric light bulb, Thomas Edison himself, felt that too much sleep was a bad thing.

Although Edison is known to have often only slept four hours a night, it is also claimed to have taken regular daytime naps as well. His average sleep seems to have been almost eight hours every 24 hours. Considering the personal philosophy of Edison, it follows that the electric light bulb was invented. No single technology has perturbed the process of human sleep as electric lights.

The healthy sleep cycle and our biological clock keeps time for the regular sleep and waking rhythm of our body. This sets a good sleep timing. Artificial light can upset the clock of our body. By registering light through the eyes, our body follows the day-night cycle. The circadian rhythm is called this daily rhythm.

We experience this rhythm every 24 hours as our earth rotates on its axis. It's the repeating cycle of 24 hours, after which our lives are patterned. Night's darkness stimulates our brain to release melatonin, the sleep hormone of the body. Melatonin helps to make people sleep. Artificial lighting decreases the release of melatonin and can affect our ability to sleep.

 the intensity of the light was not enough to disrupt the circadian rhythm of our body. Light intensity in luxury is measured. a candle gives off. Studies have shown that our biological clock can only be reset or disrupted by 180 lux. A 10-foot-distance 100-watt bulb emits 190 lux, which is enough to reset the biological clock.

Our eyes record less light with darkness. It means that our brain is producing melatonin, the sleep hormone of the body. The levels of melatonin rise higher at night and fall during the day, all in response to the light that comes into our eyes. This is how, for 1000 years, humanity has observed the day-night cycle.

Around midnight, a flashing bright light alerts your body that the sun is shining, resulting in lower levels of melatonin in your brain. This melatonin disturbance can affect the health of our sleep. It has been shown that melatonin has many health benefits of its own. Lowering your body levels can also affect our health separately from the problem of sleep. We are exposed to a lot of stress and

24/7 activity in our modern society. The combination of the two impacts our sleep severely. Sleep is no longer safe for most of us.

What's sound sleep?

Healthy sleep means you get enough sleep and experience all the stages of sleep in the right amount. How much sleep is sufficient? The opinion that adults need about eight hours a night is among sleep researchers.

A place to lie comfortably in a quiet, dark room in the middle of the day is given to research subjects. The brain waves of the volunteer are tracked to see if they go to sleep and when. The test is only 20 minutes long. A place to lie comfortably in a comfortable, dark room in the middle of the day is offered to research subjects. The brain waves of the participant are tracked to see if they go to sleep and when. The experiment is only 20 minutes long.

If a subject falls asleep in less than 5 minutes, this is a severe deficiency of sleep. The "physical and mental reactions" of these subjects are often very impaired(1). Deprived of "borderline," sleep is considered to fall asleep in 5 to 10 minutes. Sleeping between 10 and 15 minutes suggests an acceptable amount of need for sleep. Sleeping in 15 to 20 minutes or not at all suggests an excellent level of alertness for the subject.

Another way to see how you are deprived of sleep is to see how sleepy you are. The more sleep you get, the more rest you get. This measure, called the Epworth sleepiness scale(8), is correct whether you are someone that wants more or less than eight hours. You don't get enough sleep if you're tired.

The usual period of sleep.

A regular sleep cycle is the other part of getting healthy sleep. This means you're going through all the sleep cycles and experiencing each of them for a long enough time.

There are four sleeping and REM stages. Phases 1 through 4 are a progression from falling asleep (phase 1), into light sleep (phase 2) and deep sleep (phase 3 and 4). The body is in a deeply relaxed state during deep sleep. There is relaxed muscle tension, decreased blood pressure, reduced heart rate, and decreased respiration. The body secretes human growth hormone pulses during deep sleep.

Thanks to its rejuvenating properties, the human growth hormone is sometimes called the youth hormonal fountain. Your body repairs and replaces itself under human growth hormone control every night. One emerges into REM sleep after going into a deep sleep. Rapid eye movement occurs during REM sleep. REM is when we're dreaming. Researchers found that REM sleep appears to help us recall what we learned the previous day.

Why Deep Sleep is so vital to our health

What could be worse with too little or poor sleep than a few nights?

You might be more patient than most, but they can't help themselves when some people get exhausted. We can yell at anyone, and we can be blunt, impatient, and rude at times. I met a man who was always so exhausted that he told me, "I'd reason for a moment and feel my head spinning the next. I even lay down under the desk on one occasion, pretending to be searching for a plug socket so that I could close my eyes for a few seconds." He got to bed early enough most nights, but he would toss and turn all night waiting for that clock to go off in the morning. How many of us choose to live a stressful life. He has a high-pressure job, but he wasn't as successful as he needed to be by his admission, even though he worked for 15 hours. This is not as rare as you might think.

Lack of sleep was such a problem for many of the people we met during our research, so we started to investigate the subject. Why could a man go to bed tired and still take so long to get to sleep that he would wake up feeling drained instead of resting? Feedback from our weight loss customers showed us that those who slept well were more successful in weight loss and weight loss while the bad sleepers were less successful. There seemed to be some evidence that deep restorative sleep seemed to be one of the critical factors in successful weight loss and maintaining proper body weight as well as encouraging more strength, healthier responses, and more lucid thought.

We tried and helped soft music, notably Mozart. Before sleep, we tried lavender oil in the bath, and we looked at bedroom temperatures and even decoration on the pillow during sleep. Interestingly, we decided to look at beds almost as incidental to our sleep research, and that's where we made the real breakthrough. For the existing mattress, we looked at toppers and new memory foam mattresses, and they made a difference, but not enough.

Then someone recalled seeing an episode of the Tomorrow's World television program where they had carried out a thorough investigation back in the '70s into sleeping. Can you know that too? Throughout the night, they took delayed action pictures of a healthy young couple as they slept on an ordinary double bed. Then all the pictures were brought together and shown as a one-minute movie clip. It seemed the two of them were in a rave, though they had no raves back then, so it had to be a nightclub. The average person turns 60-80 times a night, with two drawbacks. First, it uses vital energy, but more importantly, it never allows enough time to restore itself to the deep sleep level that the body needs.

One day I was mentioned that we're not flat people, and yet we're trying to sleep on flatbeds all our lives. That means that our sticking out parts of our bodies leave gaps that don't touch the bed, and so small areas support the weight of our entire body. That soon hot and uncomfortable the supporting bits, and the turning process begins. We had seen flexible beds but figured they were only for hospitals or people with a disability, so we decided to look into this area more deeply.

There are plenty of adjustable beds, and the price difference is huge, so are the quality and specifications available, but let's look first at the adjustable bed principle.

The most important question before we go any further is, does it work? Okay, for most people, the short answer is' yes' most of the time. The beds shift to match the body in whatever shape it takes. By using an electrical hand control, they move into an infinite number of positions. The range of movement is impressive, you can put your feet above the level of your heart that the doctors will tell you to rest for your heart, or you can sit upright for breakfast or watch TV in bed. Best of all, you will sleep in a place where the bed fits perfectly with your body, taking all the holes and distributing your body weight throughout your whole body. This means tossing and turning much less.

You can buy ready-made beds, usually imported, which are likely to be cheaper and can be the best value for you. Or you could pay a little more and buy a bed made by hand according to your specifications. Better mattresses have a layer of memory foam over pocket springing, which allows air to circulate so that the mattress can breathe better and spread the weight to make sleep more comfortable. It makes sense to visit a showroom where you can try the mattress, or you can arrange a demonstration at home if it's difficult to get out.

Some beds may have an optional factory-installed vibration massage therapy. A good massage will penetrate the muscles and reduce tension right through the body. It can also help circulation and enhance lymphatic drainage, eliminating stress from the system that induces toxins.

With the massage on, it could be an advantage to be able to fall asleep and allow it to click off when the timer runs out. Some of them are perfectly safe to use as much as others do. Look out for any message that says "use for up to 20 minutes." Try to find someone who is accredited as a Class 2a medical device when you live in the UK and search for a signed certificate to prove it is. The forms you can buy is different from company to company, and it's a bit like buying a car or any other big product in many respects. Some firms employ salesmen who earned a poor reputation, and some were even the subject of watchdog reports. We suggest that you do your research and avoid this kind of business.

Once you consent to the final design requirements, you should be able to try a bed in your own house. Additionally, in most towns, there are specialty stores that sell a variety of flexible beds, chairs, and other similar aids. Do not feel compelled to buy the first one you see and only make a purchase if you are fully convinced that the item you are looking for will help. Looking at as many as you like and taking as long as you want to make your decision is perfectly acceptable to you. Just say no if you feel forced. If you're a pushover and you know you're not inviting a friend or relative, you know it will help you make the best choice.

Making sure the company you purchase from has been founded for more than five years can be beneficial. Some rules force a company in the UK selling therapy products to register after five years and just shut down the less reputable ones and start up again under a different name. If they have reached the threshold of five years, the likelihood of a better quality product will be improved. Everyone had to start somewhere, and if everything else looks and feels good and the promises are in place, that might be the bed for you.

Several users of such beds appear being the older generation who already live with severe pain or chronic illness and often report improved quality of life as a result of reduced or eradicated pain and increased functionality. However, they weren't the only ones benefiting, and several tight-pressure executives enjoy reduced levels of stress on adjustable beds. Even, as mentioned earlier, most professional sports people enjoy faster recovery after practice, none of us are flat people so that a bed that suits the body can be perfect for anyone.

Fail-Safe Sleep Pointers-
One is bound to work for you

It may seem like one of the biggest frustrations of life when drifting off is a struggle. It doesn't have to. Whether going to sleep is a nightmare or a pleasure, choices made all day can have a significant impact in most cases.

It is difficult for at least one in five people to get to sleep at night. For help, a small number of them consult their family physicians. Silently bear several thousand more.

In addition to being one of the most common-and troubling-of all medical problems, sleeplessness is also one of the problems with the highest number of myths.

For example, most people seem persuaded that every night they have to sleep for at least eight hours.

It's just not true. There is no correct rule as to how much we all need to sleep. Those people feel safe only when they have been sleeping for 10 hours. Others manage entirely well on 4hrs of sleep at night, like Prime Minister Margaret Thatcher.

It is also worth noting that as we get older, we all need less rest.

A second myth is that if you're having a sleepless night, you're going to have to sleep twice the next night to make up for it - and avoid damaging your health.

The truth is that if asleep just 2 hours while you're at work, the worst thing is that you'll feel tired! And the following night, you should be able to recover by having an extra few hours ' sleep thoroughly.

Many of the unlucky thousands who work night shifts could fully fix their problems if they only knew something more about the main causes of insomnia-so here are some of the reasons why people can not sleep along with the solutions.

STRESS If you go to bed thinking about the problems of the day and worrying about the things you need to sort out tomorrow, you're bound to have trouble sleeping.

Writing down your concerns will help you eradicate them from your mind. So, make a complete list of your questions. Then put the list to one side before you go to bed and spend an hour relaxing in front of the TV.

MEDICINES Pills are often prescribed to keep people awake. Sleeplessness is commonly caused by drugs used for heart disease, high blood pressure, and asthma. Ask your doctor if your prescription can be changed. Do note that 50% of people who are unable to sleep is kept because they were drinking coffee or tea last night. Caffeine is a potent stimulant. Tobacco is another possible cause of insomnia, and although a single nightcap may help you sleep, too much alcohol will certainly cause sleeplessness.

PAIN When pain keeps you awake, ask for help from your doctor. Then ask for a second option if he can't help you.

CRAMP Cramps keep up a lot of people. Use this simple exercise, and you could keep the cramp at bay. Stand one yard away from a wall barefoot. Lean forward until your hands touch the mural, but stay on the floor. Hold the position and repeat it once for 10 seconds. Do the exercise for a week three times a day and then go to bed every night.

DEPRESSION It is the depression that needs a doctor's treatment when depression and sleeplessness go together.

HUNGER If hunger keeps you awake, have a bite. There's nothing too hot, spicy, or rich. A drink of hot milk is likely to be the best. Remember, also, that you may have trouble sleeping if you're slimming. Low sugar in your blood will keep you awake. A late-night snack with very low calories could help.

NOISE Seek to soundproof your bedroom with bookshelves and double glazing if you are kept awake by the noise. And try to wear earplugs. We need to get used to it a little, but we work very well and are recommended to shift workers who have to try to sleep during the day.

Ultimately, it's worth remembering that if you're not tired, you won't be able to sleep.

If you've been grappling with all these things and still have trouble getting to sleep at night, then follow this particular bedtime scheme: calm your body thoroughly before going to bed. Take a good 10-15 minute brisk walk. Talk about the issues of your day and write down all your thoughts in a journal. Hold it by your side and write it down any time you get a new problem in your brain.

Have a 15-minute quiet, hot tub.

Go to sleep with a book or magazine that is soothing. Try to keep your bedtime reading comfortable. And have a book available to spare.

Close your eyes as you turn off the light and try to transfer yourself somewhere stunning, soothing, and hot somewhere. Imagine lying alone on a calm, sunny beach, for example. Try to hear the shore waves and the high overhead sound of seagulls.

This easy program is likely to send you in minutes to bed. But if you can't sleep, don't think about lying there. Get up, sit down, and reread your book in a comfortable chair. Make a hot, milky drink for yourself. So, when you start yawning, go back to bed.

On a web search drive for Wellness, there are millions of hits-from psychological to cardiac fitness, physical health, yoga, cancer, how to solve both those ailments such as hypertension, diabetes, stoke, weight loss, and obesity tips, and how to grow taller, with many other ideas being honored. Having any place which has so much to give on all these fronts requires quite a bit of research, let alone one that can balance all the needs for your innermost well-being-joy, peace, and more. Sake of wellness, you could learn to look out and end up taking yourself several time, a kind of one-stop-shop

CHAPTER THREE

Sleep - The Reason, The Purpose and How to Get It

Researchers have discovered many times in many fields, the purpose of sleeping and why we sleep, but none overlap their fields to put together the studies. Research on sleep, pillows, electronics, blood flow, chiropractic, massage therapy, brain basics, and several other health fields took about 15 years to understand that sleep is essential for our health and why. Sleep is a necessary need for survival. As one author concluded, "the animals were not harmed by lack of sleep because they all died from organ failure."

Looking at data analysis, we get that, as we are human animals, we would die of organ failure without sleep. Sleep must, therefore, have a healing effect on the organs of the body. Our organs begin to shut down without sleep, and we develop a disease; get sick. When you consult with a lot of people who are not sleeping well, you will find that they are often sick and on medications.

Some current studies indicate how we feel and act as if drugged or drunk without sleep. We see how the body works by observing the body structure and skeleton through studies of MDs, chiropractic, and massage therapy. Brain studies showed that chemicals were produced by the brain to heal the body. It also claimed that the brain uses 20 percent of our overall blood flow, and 50 percent of the blood oxygen is used. This research gave me a glimpse of another high blood pressure cause. Muscle research shows that the muscles of the neck contract around the arteries, restricting the blood flow to the brain under pressure.

Recent studies into how our anatomy functions show that all electrical contact from and to the brain passes through the neck area and the spinal column. Through brain research, we find that the brain controls all functions of the body, muscles, nerves, and even gives us the energy needed to move. The brain consumes and uses more than 400,000,000 bits of information per second, minute, hour, weekly. If it functions at full when alive, when would the brain have time to heal our body? If we could reduce the intake, maybe the brain will be able to heal us with some energy?

Research in many areas of health show that the body repairs itself, and the only time the energy is available during sleep.

The object of sleep is to maintain a healthy body!

Over 50% of the input signals stop relieving up the energy needed to heal our body during sleep. The body fights infections during sleep, heals, rejuvenates, and defrags the electrical information, freeing up the next day's storage space. Sleep helps our bodies to be healed through brain time and energy. During this period, any restriction of energy or blood flow to or from the brain would stop or reduce brain healing.

A pillow enters the picture of the bed. There are two ways the brain can be affected by a restriction; blood flow and electrical flow. For proper blood flow, the neck muscles must be relaxed, and the neck vertebra must be open so that electrons can flow freely to and from the brain.

Support (pillow) must support the weight of the head while relaxing the muscles of the neck, keeping the neck in alignment on the back or side. Aligning the spine while sleeping allows all parts of the body to be reached by the healing. The pillow is an essential part of getting good deep sleep as a Chinese emperor who demanded and received the perfect sleep support over 5,000 years ago, even though he slept on a wooden surface.

The pillow of today should adhere to a comfortable mattress while supporting the weight of the head and maintaining alignment of the chest. To fit their body structure and way of sleeping, side, or back, each person must be measured for a size pillow.

Just as we buy clothes in sizes, we can now buy our pillows n sizes to fit our sleeping method. A company has found a way to calculate the sleep triangle of people and create five pillow sizes to match everyone. Side sleepers select by crossing their body structure to their height from the side sleeping chart — the same with the back-sleeping map of back sleepers.

The company has refined deep sleep to a pillow's proper size and shape. Even after what the pillow did, they named their company; (Align-Right) aligns the neck at night.

It takes a pillow for deep sleep. Our quality of life requires good deep sleep. Deep sleep is needed overnight, or we're going to die early. All we do revolves around how well we're sleeping, not how long, but more research and a different story: proper sleep and a good life.

Sleep-Recovery Aid Forgotten

If the weight training bug has bitten you, sleep may be the last thing in your mind. You probably have devoured all the reading materials that teach you how to tear down muscle cells efficiently. In reality, for this type of constructive self-torture, you're searching for new methods. In fact, after a workout, you may be mentally chastising yourself, thinking about ways you have missed to harm muscle fibers better. What's not killing you, does it make you stronger? You may very well be one of the savants on the subject of supplementation who would walk into whatever supermarket and contend with the resident bodybuilder employee, whether arginine or leucine is better for protein synthesis. But are you investing in the one aid for recovery that doesn't cost you a dime?

Substituting your weight training with far more relaxation may be one of the most underestimated techniques you could use to help you recover from those thrashing exercises of the Central Nervous System (CNS) that you say you always do. If you could invent a pill-shaped supplement that could improve the performance of the exercise, restore and dissipate the effects of stress and exhaustion, and strengthen the immune system, you'd make a million dollars overnight. How about having a few more sleeping clinks?

As they age, we usually sleepless is it because the pineal gland produces less melatonin in our brain. Among the contributing factors to muscle wasting (sarcopenia) is the lack of sleep among seniors. It's also true that as we mature, the hypophysis releases less growth hormone. The growth hormone is substantially produced as we sleep. Is this a matter for the chick or the egg? Is it inevitable that we must accept hormonal declines as we go along, or maybe we need to get plenty of sleep?

Whether you're twenty-something, the truth is that if you miss a lot of sleep, you may have more in common with an octogenarian. This may lose your technological edge and might even gain muscle mass. Not only can this be in debt to a financial creditor, but you can also be in debt to your body because you owe it a lot of sleep. This is often referred to as "sleep debt," and it's not just about catching up on weekends for a few more hours. Not only does bed debt go down. This accumulates over time and needs to be paid for. And just as it takes time to gather, paying it off also takes time. Getting one or two extra hours a night will help this gradually.

As they age, we usually sleepless is it because the pineal gland produces less melatonin in our brain. Among the contributing factors to muscle wasting (sarcopenia) is the lack of sleep among seniors. It's also true that as we mature, the hypophysis releases less growth hormone. The growth hormone is substantially produced as we sleep. Is this a matter for the chick or the egg? Is it inevitable that we must accept hormonal declines as we go along, or maybe we need to get plenty of sleep?

Whether you're twenty-something, the truth is that if you miss a lot of sleep, you may have more in common with an octogenarian. This may lose your technological edge and might even gain muscle mass. Not only can this be in debt to a financial creditor, but you can also be in debt to your body because you owe it a lot of sleep. This is often referred to as "sleep debt," and it's not just about catching up on weekends for a few more hours. Not only does bed debt go down. This accumulates over time and needs to be paid for. And just as it takes time to gather, paying it off also takes time. Getting one or two extra hours a night will help this gradually.

Some Sleep Facts: Every night, you sleep in full cycles. Everyone sleeps in cycles of 90 minutes. There are five parts to a cycle, but let's break it down to three:

• You've got 65 minutes of normal sleep first. This is also called deep sleep, non-REM, or slow-wave sleep (SWS). To this stage of sleep, there is a strong parasympathetic component of the nervous system (healing). During this stage, there is usually no dreaming.

• Twenty minutes of REM (rapid eye movement) sleep in the second stage. This is when you're dreaming. During REM sleep, the muscles also tend to be paralyzed.

• There are another 5 minutes of non-REM sleep in the final and third phase.

During deep sleep, growth hormone has been studied to be secreted during the first (heavy parasympathetic) stage. Here there is a reciprocal relationship; not only does deeper sleep produce higher growth hormone levels, but more growth hormone appears to cause more in-depth and longer sleep stages.

Sleep Repairs the Stress Effects There is something called a "multiple latency test for sleep" (MSLT). This shows that the faster you fall asleep, the sleeper you are (that is, the more you need to sleep). Those subjects deprived of sleep over some time are showing increasing signs of daily fatigue. The more nights they go to bed without performance, the more they get tired. They get depressed and less alert. This condition can be changed slowly by having someone under an 8-hour or more - a-night sleep regimen.

The longer you get tired, the longer it takes to recover from a workout. Something is called the dual-factor theory of rehabilitation. It states that after a hard workout, two components are present. One's level of fitness is increased as well as one's level of fatigue. Emotional stress and a lack of sleep can also affect the fatigue element. Too little sleep can result in a state of exhaustion that can hinder your progress significantly.

Sleep Improves the glutamine overdosage of the immune system? To enhance recovery, many bodybuilders ingest vast amounts of glutamine. While there are some evidence to suggest that after physiological trauma such as surgery or burning patients, massive quantities boost the immune system, there is little evidence to prove that the usual weight trainer is getting any increased benefit. For better sleep, wounds heal quicker. Research with rats indicates that white blood cell count is decreased by sleep deprivation. More extended periods of sleep lead to higher numbers of white blood cells and higher immune function. You may not immediately want to chop the glutamine, but at least try to sleep more. The effects of deep healthy sleep, as well as adequate food and hydration, can be sufficient for recovery.

Some methods for a Better Night's Sleep

• Do not practice less than 3 hours before bedtime. If you do, your heart rate will be higher than if you did not come during the first few hours of sleep. Also, the harder you exercise, the more you will require non-REM or deep sleep.

• Before bedtime, drinks a glass of warm milk or tea.

• Make the room as dark as you could, or wear one of those eye-catching sleeping masks.

• Don't eat before you go to bed. DO NOT take pills for sleep.

• If you don't count goats, you might want to use a transistor radio. Set it to low volume and add earbuds to your ears. This "white noise" is going to go on and on, so you're going to drift off to sleep.

• Write down a to-dodo list before going to bed if you have a busy schedule the next day. This can give you some psychological peace of mind rather than worrying and planning to lie in bed.

The relationship between normal sleepers and exercise is not all that many studies. Maybe this is because research requires money and is an activity that is not usually engaged in unless there is some possible outcome of monetary increase; there is not much profit just telling someone to sleep more.

Finally, psychologists strive to become more concerned about the risk of the exercise of sleep disorders like sleep apnea, but no one agrees that only a full night's sleep is good. May not hesitate to seek advice with a competent medical practitioner if you have persistent sleep problems.

How to Succeed in Life if you Sleep Less and hav e more Energy

We all believe in the myth that for seven to eight hours a day, we have to sleep compulsorily. That's not at all necessary. We should recognize that our sleep quality is more important than the length of time we sleep for. For many reasons, many people want to sleep less. Some people may have a lot of work and may wish to extra hours to finish their work. Many people may not be able to sleep or lay on the floor and not sleep for them, and so on. But as we've all been led to believe we need seven or eight hours of sleep, we're just lying on our beds and continuing to worry about our work. We can't sleep well, and we can't get up and do our work. The effect is that we feel drowsy throughout the next day, have neck pain, and are therefore not going to be able to function with concentration. Research has shown that if we have about four to five hours of quality sleep, that's enough for us to feel fresh and energetic. To get such a quality-sleep, you can follow a few steps to gain more energetic hours. If you get these extra hours, you'll be able to accomplish more.

The first thing you ought to remember is that insomnia has never caused anyone to die. But if we're worried about something and don't sleep, because of our worries, our energy and resistance levels drop, and we may be affected by infections. The inference, therefore, is that the concerns take a toll, not sleeplessness.

Another argument we must consider is that sleeping is primarily two phases. The first is the phase of a deep sleep, and the second is the sleep of the Rapid Eye Movement (REM). When we have a deep sleep, the blood does the job of repairing by flowing through all of our body parts, muscles, and cells. Memory processes are set correctly and organized correctly in the REM stage. We only get dreams in this level. It's not that we've got deep sleep or REM sleep all the time. Alternatively, we get both. After a day's work, when we retire for bed and fall asleep, we get deep sleep. Then comes the sleep of the REM. It will be longer for both the deep sleep and REM sleep we undergo shortly after bed retirement in the evenings. Whatever kind of sleep we get is going to be shorter after that.

The melatonin levels in our body determine the duration of our sleep. Melatonin is a hormone that is formed in the daytime in our body, and the primary source for this is sunlight. When the day comes to an end after the sunset, this chemical will be released from the body, and we will sleep when the chemical comes out of our system. We should, therefore, increase the levels of melatonin in our body that we should go out for about an hour in sunlight. The early morning sun and the evening sunlight are particularly useful. When we move around during the peak noons, the sun's UV rays can affect us. Spending an hour in the sunshine keeps proper levels of melatonin, which gives us a good sleep.

When the body temperature drops, we feel sleepy immediately. That's what's going on during nights, and even the heart rate and blood pressure are going down. The brain thinks it should trigger sleep when these happen. So, we should do our daily exercises to avoid such a fall in body temperature. We will sleep better because of these workouts, which will increase our energy levels.

Similarly, it logically transmits a message to the brain when we are surrounded by darkness that sleep must be triggered. So, sleeping in the dark is suitable for having a deep and better sleep.

Another perfect way to get more energy despite less sleep is to walk in the sun as soon as we get up in the morning. Sunlight gives us the energy we need, and because our brain is fully activated, we feel fresh.

We were advised to follow a strict routine or time-table to have a better sleep. If we go to sleep every day at the same hour, we can sleep better and enjoy higher levels of energy. If we go through irregular hours, the brain becomes confused, so the sleep we get may not be of good quality.

During the day, we can also have power naps, but we should make sure they don't exceed 30 minutes. Another advice given by experts is that it can promote better sleep if we have a cup of warm milk before we retire to bed. Reducing the intake of coffee, tea, and alcohol is a significant step that if we want to sleep better, we should never ignore it.

When the body temperature drops, we feel sleepy immediately. That's what's going on during nights, and even the heart rate and blood pressure are going down. The brain thinks it should trigger sleep when these happen. So, we should do our daily exercises to avoid such a fall in body temperature. We will sleep better because of these workouts, which will increase our energy levels.

Similarly, it logically transmits a message to the brain when we are surrounded by darkness that sleep must be triggered. So, sleeping in the dark is suitable for having a deep and better sleep.

Another perfect way to get more energy despite less sleep is to walk in the sun as soon as we get up in the morning. Sunlight gives us the energy we need, and because our brain is fully activated, we feel fresh.

We were advised to follow a strict routine or time-table to have a better sleep. If we go to sleep every day at the same hour, we can sleep better and enjoy higher levels of energy. If we go through irregular hours, the brain becomes confused, so the sleep we get may not be of good quality.

During the day, we can also have power naps, but we should make sure they don't exceed 30 minutes. Another advice given by experts is that it can promote better sleep if we have a cup of warm milk before we retire to bed. Reducing the intake of coffee, tea, and alcohol is a significant step that if we want to sleep better, we should never ignore it.

Clear Conscious is the Best Sleeping Pill

Rest is one of life's most essential needs. That living being needs to sleep to survive. Understanding that there is no scientific reason why we need to sleep is extremely interesting. Yet we all know that a healthy living needs rest. If we don't even get a night's sleep, we won't be able to do our daily work reasonably. If we don't have five days of sleep, we can start hallucinating. It would be difficult for anyone to stay awake after a while.

Having a good sleep is now considered one of the main health and longevity factors. Research by Pennsylvania State University found that losing sleep can affect hormone levels and create harmful chemicals in the body. They also concluded that it is because they are better sleepers that women live longer than men for several years.

Nevertheless, due to their so-called modern lifestyle and their desire to obtain more material benefits in this country, many people find it extremely difficult to get sound sleep. As the modern world seems to value wealth and power more than anything else in the world, people are often willing to do anything to make it richer and more powerful. Yet most of these men end up losing sleep given all the comforts they've acquired through their wealth strength.

There is something that hampers the sleep in gaining excessive wealth and power. Those who respect sleep realize that no material possession is necessary to deny to all human beings the sleep that nature provides.

The Importance of Sleep We all understand that the loss of sleep in the night is one of the consequences of doing wrong in our life. In their air-conditioned rooms in their luxurious beds, a criminal and immoral person passes through the sleepless night while a man who clears conscious sleeps without a bed and a fan even in the hot weather. A man who doesn't get a good night's sleep soon gets afflicted with many body and mind ailments and soon pays a heavy price for his sleeplessness.

It's better to lose a million dollars than a good night's sleep." Let's find out the connection between sound sleep and a person's consciousness?

Four Stages of Reality A person has four stages of consciousness in the Indian scriptures of "Madukya Upanishad," i.e., 1. The phase of waking up 2. The phase of the dreams, 3. The stage of deep sleep and 4. A man perceives the world through his senses, i.e., through his eyes, ears, nose, tongue, and skin, in the waking stage. A man perceives the world through his mind in the dream stage as all his senses are inactive in the dream stage while his mind remains active. The senses and mind are dormant in a deep sleep, and the man has no sense of time. Through his religious identity, the man's physical integrity is subsumed.

The final stage of consciousness is described as "Turia," in which man enters the state of pure consciousness or divinity. This stage was defined in yoga as the stage of Samadhi, whose glimpses during meditation and yoga are possible.

The four stages of consciousness can be contrasted with the four stages of nature mentioned in scriptures, i.e., body, mind, soul, and Spirit (God). This is different from the scientist's interpretation of reality, which beliefs in just one reality, i.e., body. They believe that the thoughts in mind are due to the bio-chemical that the body produces and therefore have no independent existence other than the body.

Therefore, the four sages of knowledge can be associated as viewed in scriptures with the four stages of truth. The deep sleep here corresponds to the soul's reality. If the mind is disturbed, it is impossible to attain deep sleep.

The Importance of Sleep In scriptures, the mystery of the soul is well-founded. It is considered the root of the body, mind, and ego. Therefore, when we are in a deep sleep, the individual's soul is fused with the infinite soul and derives from this union the infinite intellectual. The soul achieves its equilibrium due to this union, which is lost in the everyday practice of life. The mastered soul makes the body and mind perfect because our body and mind are the mirrors of the soul. Therefore, when a man wakes up after deep sleep in the morning, he feels fresh, and all his body stresses and tiredness are gone. The deeper the ailment, the longer it takes to sleep to compensate for the damage to the body and mind.

Nonetheless, deep sleep is the scientists ' most enigmatic. "Why do we need so much sleep? It describes as one of science's greatest mysteries. Nevertheless, the scientists have no question about the benefits of deep sleep that are mentioned in the following words:- The value of sleep is not fully understood. What we know is that sleep is a cycle that is anabolic or constructing. And we assume this recovers the energy supplies of the body that have been exhausted by the events of the day.

Sleep is also the time when most of the body's repair work is done; muscle tissue is healed and repaired. We know, for instance, that during sleep growth hormone is secreted. This hormone is essential for children's growth but is also necessary for tissue reconstruction throughout adulthood.

Our soul's function is the source of infinite wisdom that has existed in the universe since it was created as part of the eternal Universal Soul or God. This wisdom is used by the mind to solve new and novel problems. Through the use of the local knowledge gained in this life and the soul's infinite wisdom, all unanswered life issues are discussed in mind. Man often by keeping himself occupied in day-to-day jobs prevents these problems. Nevertheless, as he tries to sleep at night, these things haunt his mind, and it is not possible to avoid a conversation between the soul and the rational brain. Such talks will proceed until a solution has been found.

Our soul is capable of solving any problems in our lives that upset us. Nevertheless, the soul can not solve the problems that arise due to defying the conscious as the soul can not go against its essential nature. Thus it is impossible to resolve the conflict between the soul and the mind, and the soul can never rest in peace.

While a bored body can conserve its damage and lost energy tissue through sound sleep, and the troubled mind can achieve peace and tranquility through proper sleep, the guilty conscious finds no relief as his soul can not rescue the man. The result is sleeplessness that no medicinal products can cure. The damage caused by such insomnia is durable and irreversible.

Sleep is invaluable. Because of its role in keeping the body and mind safe, the importance of sound sleep can not be overestimated. While nature has been kind in granting both men and women the gift of sleep with a clear consciousness, it takes away the sleep of those whose consciousness is uncertain. Compared to the damage done to him due to the lack of sleep induced by nature to a man going against his conscience, the benefits gained by the individual by going against his conscious are nothing. If a person keeps his consciousness pure and dry, for a healthy and happy life, he does not need medication.

CHAPTER FOUR

How to Lose Weight While You Sleep

Most of us take sleep as a matter of course. We're supposed to need our "rest" without worrying a lot about it. Yet sleep's most crucial function is to regenerate our bodies. Our muscles, ligaments, skin, cartilage, and other working parts of our body are worn down in the process if we participate in muscle-taxing or physical exercise work throughout the day. To reconstruct these damaged parts, the body needs a time of rest. That's what's going on during sleep.

In other words, during sleep, the body embarks on a restorative cycle. And this recovery process uses energy to restore lean muscle mass as well as different body tissue types. This is worth repeating— the means of reconstruction that occur during sleep use fuel. And if the restorative processes operate smoothly and efficiently, the energy required comes from the places in our body where our fat cells store energy.

So while we sleep the repairs of the body and regenerate the tissue of the muscles, ligaments, tendons, and lean muscle by eating the calories that we eat during the day, and if that's not enough, excess fat will be consumed.

There is many thing worth noting about this operation. They have an essential role to play in how it works effectively.

Collagen is the essential protein found in our bodies for the body repair process. It is the main component of our hair, teeth, bones, cartilage, and connective tissue and can be found in all the organs of our body. Cartilages are the cushion and shock absorber between joints, which is why we remain flexible and mobile. But the very things that break down during our normal daily activities are cartilage and other soft body tissues. So the body is continually regenerating healthy cartilage and other soft tissue, and this cycle, which relies on a steady source of collagen, helps to keep us young and flexible.

Unfortunately, as we grow old, our bodies lose the ability to produce collagen at enough levels to support the therapeutic processes, our bodies are designed to perform. This can be a significant contributor to a prematurely aged look and can have a substantial impact on our strength and mobility.

It is, therefore, appropriate for a collagen supplement to be paired with other natural ingredients to have a dramatic impact on deep restorative processes that occur during sleep. This, in turn, can give more energy to the body, build more lean muscle, and burn more fat.

Amino acids enhance the process of regeneration. The process of reconstruction also depends on a unique combination of amino acids found in collagen. Such particular amino acids, based on collagen, help to retain lean muscle mass as part of the restoration process and allow the body to absorb fat for energy more readily while the long therapeutic sleep cycles. This normal metabolic component contributes directly to weight loss and our ability to keep our "right" weight.

But again, as we age, collagen development is decreased in our body and its particular amino acids. The natural ingredient L-Carnitine can significantly improve the natural function of the body to turn excess fat into readily available energy when combined adequately with collagen in a natural supplement. This unique amino acid combination works as a native "turbocharger" during deep sleep to help your body rebuild, restore, and create lean muscle while burning stored excess fat to provide the energy needed.

It is vital not to eat before bed because the body uses deep sleep for the restoration process; it is essential not to eat until three hours before going to sleep when using a collagen supplement. This is because we do not want the competition of nutrients between undigested food and the unique nutrient formula of the collagen supplement. If the body has to deal with digestion, the collagen solution will not be fully absorbed. Therefore, while you sleep, your body will not perform its natural restorative process, but will be concerned with unprocessed foods and will store fat from the ongoing digestive process instead of burning fat as the energy for deep sleep restorative process.

It tends to put us in a "frustrative diet" loop. The less time the body spends in deep, restful sleep (without opposing digestion), the less energy it requires to recover its natural health, and the less fat it consumes to help this natural healing cycle.

Now we know that our overall health always goes hand in hand with deep, restful sleep and weight loss.

During the deep restorative sleep cycle, reducing or eliminating food intake three hours before bedtime allow body to use its natural fat reserves for metabolic fuel.

Building on this process, collagen weight loss products Natural collagen supplements allow the natural process to help people lose weight and become healthier naturally. For example, L-Carnitine, Aloe Barbadensis (Aloe Vera) and a mixture of Collagen is the product called Lose and Snooze. The Collagen leads to a more youthful look, greater flexibility, and all-round agility and energy.

The collagen supplement enhances the deep sleep needed to enable the normal metabolic functions of your body to take place, like when we were children. L-Carnitine, the second component, facilitates the burning of fat in favor of natural regeneration, a therapeutic process that takes place during deep sleep. Aloe Vera(Aloe Barbadensis) contains numerous nutrients and amino acids that support the ability of your body to create its collagen to create a healthy environment.

Many collagen supplement users, such as Lose and Snooze, reported good results. But researchers stress that an integral part of therapy is going to bed on an empty stomach. Most users report using just a connective tissue method in mixture with an empty stomach before bedtime has benefited their overall health and helped them lose weight naturally.

And since cartilage supplements only help to lose excess fat (while muscle reconstruction), they can be used by anyone— not just people who want to lose weight. They have also benefited people that wish to prefer better sleep, retrofit lean muscle, strengthen the image, and redefine their bodies while keeping a healthy weight.

Secrets for better Sleep that have been Scientifically Proven

We've been spending at least one-quarter of our lives. The body and mind are rejuvenated by sleep. It is critical for health to have a good night's sleep. But as necessary, most people can't sleep well in this century.

Here I will share in deep sleep ten scientifically proven secrets.

1. Stick to a schedule of sleep: people hate living on a schedule, but it is essential for work productivity. The same also applies to the human body. We have an internal clock telling the body when to wake up and sleep, and it doesn't like being continuously reset. It was easy for our ancestors to adhere to a sleep schedule when

there was no power and bright lights, but we have to make it a routine for us. You are spared from heart disease, stroke, diabetes, and even cancer by a regular sleep schedule.

How to set a schedule for sleep? Some, like me, have tried without success. What I've found is that you have to teach yourself through a series of routines like you train your dog to tell your body it's time to sleep. Before sleep, some examples are listening to music and taking a hot shower. If you maintain this pattern for at least one week, your body will learn and program to your sleep schedule itself (better than a Nest thermostat).

2. Remove lights. Lights inhibit melatonin production, a sleep-triggering hormone. Light deceives our brain into thinking it's time to wake up, so soon, a person who sleeps with lights on is less likely to sleep. It's not just bright lights, and it can affect sleep even in small amounts of light. Make a habit to turn off all lights before you go to bed to avoid lights. Even nightlights should be avoided if possible. Keep a small flashlight if you're in the habit of waking up at night. Try to get some sunshine during the day; people working in offices are much less exposed to sunlight, so their brain won't be able to differentiate that between your night light. The result? You're already alive.

3. Avoid devices. Needless to say, it's mobile phones and tablets that keep people staying late. It's a bad idea to check your email before bed, both because it's backlit and keeps your mind busy. Most electronic devices ' type of light is close to sunlight and keeps your brain awake. If it is essential to check your laptop or mobile in bed, try to reduce as much as possible its brightness.

4. Remove noise, or even interrupt unexpected or noisy noises. Such unwelcome sounds can quickly disturb deep sleep also if you

manage to go to bed. What's the best solution, then? Using plugs for the mouth! But I should warn that this is not the best option, as some sounds can improve sleep. The sounds of' white' and' pink' encourage restful sleep. White sounds are a distorted mix of different frequency sounds, while' pink noise' is a mix of constant frequency sounds. But if you can't avoid other sounds, the best option is to use earplugs.

5. Stay in a more relaxed place. High temperature tends to keep our cycles of metabolism more involved while a low temperature (more comfortable than your daytime) keeps them to a minimum. The brain produces a hormone called melatonin that allows you to sleep at lower temperatures. Wearing minimum clothes and selecting natural fabrics increases the circulation of air and lowers body temperature and helps you fall asleep more quickly.

6. Keep exercises at a minimum if you don't go to the gym a couple of hours before bedtime. Exercises keep your heart rate and other metabolic activities high, so you're going to have trouble sleeping. You can calm your body and help it slow down by taking a hot bath before bedtime.

7. Doesn't alcohol allow us to sleep more quickly and better? Think again. Alcohol affects our brain and nervous system; we will feel relaxed and tired, but the more profound state of sleep will be disturbed. So if you're planning to drink, do it a couple of hours before bedtime. And make sure you have plenty of water to drink.

8. Smoking cuts too. Unlike alcohol, nicotine is a stimulant; it helps you stay awake, just like caffeine. Stop smoking, this is the best for you, or make sure you stay between your last puff and sleep time for many hours.

9. Eat foods rich in carbohydrates that improve sleep. While eating a heavy meal near your sleep time is not healthy, you can always eat a snack. And from your snack list, avoid protein-rich foods, they can keep you awake.

10. That's wrong. Holding a calm mind always represents our feelings on our skin. The body will have a hard time relaxing if you're tensed or nervous. Keeping your tools and working away from the house is the best way to avoid worries.

I trained myself to follow each of the secrets mentioned above and give me a deep morning sleep and refreshment. Practice and see the miracles happen for at least seven days.

The bond for both migraines and problems with sleep respiration

The recent revelation by Michelle Bachmann that she is suffering from migraines raises an essential point that most doctors and the lay public do not appreciate: the importance of proper night breathing. Sleep deprivation is widely known to cause or aggravate migraines, but what is generally believed is that migraine patients sleep well at night. I can make a convincing argument that all migraine sufferers have some variation of a sleep-breathing disorder, only a small fraction of which has obstructive sleep apnea.

Not Your Standard Migraines Classic migraine headaches are described as one-sided, painful, pounding, severe headaches combined with nausea, vomiting, light, or sensitivity to sound. Note that migraines are getting better with sleep, usually.

Neurologists have recently expanded the definition of a migraine attack. Whenever the nerves become over-sensitive and overly excitable in any part of your body, you will experience symptoms unique to that part of your body.

For example, if the nerve endings are unexpectedly extra sensitive in your sinuses, then you will feel pressure, nasal congestion, pain and post-nasal drip. Besides, it has been shown that, with regular CAT scans, the vast majority of a chronic sinus headache and pain sufferers may have a migraine variation. Most individuals are empirically put on oral antibiotics when there is no contamination of bacteria.

You can also have your stomach migraines. This may occur as nausea, vomiting, diarrhea, constipation, or bloating. Kids suffering from chronic abdominal pain have been speculated to suffer from migraines potentially.

If you have a migraine attack in your internal ears, you will experience dizziness, lightheadedness, feeling fullness, hearing loss, and ringing. This is considered the migraine vestibular type.

Problems Because of your language?

The minimal size of their upper airways, particularly in the space behind the tongue and in the nose, is an anatomical characteristic that we see all migraineurs have in common. We're talking about how most modern humans have smaller jaws and facial skeletons because our diets and lifestyles have changed radically. This results in dental crowding, which narrows the room behind your tongue, mainly when you're lying flat on your back. You'll stop breathing and you'll wake up to turn to your side or belly when you go into a deep sleep while your muscles relax. This is why most people on their backs can't sleep with this sort of anatomy.

Are you A What?

Generally, these breathing delays are not long enough to be considered apneas (at least 10-second pauses) and usually do not result in lower levels of oxygen. It does, however, lead to more frequent excitement and fragmentation of sleep. You can't stay in a deep sleep, permanently. You won't even realize that you are waking up in most cases. What you're going to feel isn't refreshed when you wake up in the morning or feel like you've only been sleeping for 2-3 hours.

A new type of sleep-breathing problem was identified in the early 1990s, called the upper airway resistance syndrome (UARS). Young women and men who did not meet official requirements of obstructive sleep apnea were recruited and were subjected to testing of esophageal stress. What they showed was a gradual increase in negative inspiratory pressures that led to exciting, but not severe or prolonged to be called hypopneas or apneas. Officially, apneas request at least 10 seconds of respiratory delays, while hypopneas require an airflow fall of 30 to 50 percent, along with arousals and decreases in oxygen levels. However, if apneas or hypopneas don't reach the 10-second threshold, they won't be scored at all. By principle, therefore, you can stop breathing 20 to 30 times an hour and not have technically obstructive apnea for sleep.

Being unable deep to get , refreshing sleep could lead to a physiological stress state, where your whole nervous system could become hypersensitive and heightened, even transferring into the daytime. Low quality of sleep often causes muscle stress and stretching that may predispose to headaches, TMJ, spasms of the neck, and backaches. Even your senses could become sensitive overly, especially to changes in the environment, chemical, fragrance, or odor. Also, your imagination and intuition can be enhanced in this main situation.

Note how many of the symptoms of a migraine attack are very close to those of a hangover: vomiting, nausea, bright lights and brain fog, and loud noises resistance. This is your unconscious nervous system that over-reacts to something that is not ordinarily upsetting.

Clear steps to take So if you have any of these forms of migraine, what can you do apart from taking prescription medicines? For better sleep and less headaches, here are five necessary steps:

1. Between 3-4 hours before bedtime, do not eat anything. Your stomach juices can promote reflex in your throat, causing more excitement and less efficient sleep.

2. Within 3-4 hours of bedtime, do not drink alcohol. Alcohol relaxes the muscles of your neck, creating more frequent blockages and anticipation.

3. Keep clear of your nose. If, for whatever reason, your nose is stuffy, do everything you can to keep it open. A stuffy nose produces a downstream vacuum effect in the throat, which causes the tongue to fall back more often. Using nasal nasal dilator strips,

saline irrigation systems, decongestants, allergy drugs, and even surgery if the previous solutions are not working well.

4. Don't lie on the back. Due to gravity, back sleeping encourages the collapse of the tongue.

5. Help relax the nervous system, do more yoga, tai chi, and deep breathing exercises. Take 4-5 deep breaths whenever you have 15 to 30 seconds, such as standing in line, holding one on the phone, or walking to another room, between significant activities. It helps stimulate the parasympathetic nervous system, helping to calm and relax the body. It can also assist with acupuncture.

Once you have explored these cautious methods and want to bring them to the next level, consider conducting a thorough evaluation of your eyes, nose, and throat to see that you have no narrowing in your breathing passages. The doctor will concentrate in general on your nasal septum and turbinates, tonsils, adenoids, the nostrils (to see if they collapse), soft palate, lingual tonsils, and base areas of the tongue.

There will be either UARS or sleep apnea for many people with migraines. Standard treatment services can substantially help to relieve migraines. Additionally, dental implants or advanced orthodontics are excellent option-these solutions are more critical if you have any significant dental crowding, bite problems, or a tiny mouth. Dentists can also assist with TMJ, which can significantly interfere with migraines and other syndromes of facial pain.

Botox may also be used for migraines, but just like prescription migraine medicines, it only covers the causes instead of treating them.

To some extent, OTC drugs and natural herbs and supplements (like feverfew) are not benefiting everyone while they function in different degrees. But if you're interested, it's worth trying.

Food causing migraines: red wine, aged cheeses, candy, and MSG.

I usually don't recommend surgery, but if more conventional options don't work, it can be a viable option. There are several different choices, depending on where the breathing pathways are narrowing.

Hope for Migraine Sufferers One of the most rewarding experiences is having patients tell me that after various forms of surgery, their migraines (or even headaches of the cluster) went away. With some of the non-surgical, conservative options, it also happens sometimes.

Migraines need to be handled with a pill in our society, and I want to refute the misconception. I comprehend that the best way to treat migraines is to strive to achieve the best possible sleep (by breathing better). To help you breathe and sleep better, it is essential to combine the different conservative steps with techniques. Maybe instead of focusing solely on migraines, it's far more necessary to m actually-evaluate your complete life circumstance and be willing to make lifestyle changes that could not only enhance your migraines but also develop your quality of life significantly.

Your immune system wants too much rest!

People who catch cold can recover faster and even avoid catching a cold in the first place in some cases as long as they help their bodies improve their immunity. There are some popular ways to improve the self-defense system, and some interesting approaches are less apparent to us. For instance, it inflames your nasal passages when you inhale a cold virus. The cycle of inflammation causes the body to release chemicals, including histamine. You are at a greater risk of catching a cold or a virus when you have a weak immune system. Your immune system is responsible to help you fight infections; thus, it can not function properly if your immune system is nervous.

Sleep apnea can have serious health consequences and has been associated with problems such as heart failure, stroke, high blood pressure, and diabetes. Obstructive sleep apnea causes frequent breathing delays that happen when the muscles relax while sleeping, causing soft tissue to collapse in the back of the throat and blocking the upper airway. Several clinical trials have shown that regular exercise is closely associated with increased immunity, with a focus on daily use.

This body temperature trend will result in poor sleep if you stay inactive, which will stop you from sleeping deeply. Nearing stress management by a health and fitness strategy to wellness can give you "bank money" when it comes to preventing stress, when it happens, it can give you the energy you need to deal with stress. The previous elements form part of a health and fitness lifestyle approach. The authors suggested that restoring sleep is a critical component of medical therapy and an essential preventive measure. Such results were illustrated by several studies, the latest published in Sleep Bulletin's previous issue, that indicate that adequate sleep is correlated with a decreased risk of mortality in the general population.

They're not gaining much, but they're losing a lot of their wellbeing, you can see it in their social interactions, their ability to learn and think clearly. Sleep is among the keys to a proper diet and a healthy lifestyle. The topic of constant study is other public health risks such as poor nutrition, cigarettes, excess alcohol, and lack of exercise. On the flip side, little research on the specific topic of sleep was done.

Step 1 is sleeping softly. Perhaps you witnessed this in college during boring lectures. Your body is barely asleep, your eyes are moving slightly, and you are quickly awakened, usually with a startled "jump." You will often have dream-like visions during this point.

Step 2 is when your eyes stop moving, and your brain waves start slowing down.

Stage 3 starts deep sleep as very slow brain waves, known as delta waves, take over faster brain waves, known as sleep spindles.

Stage 4 is a deep state in which all movements of the muscle stops. During this state, it is hard to be revived, and when you are, you are often in a dizzy, disoriented condition.

Five is named sleeping REM (rapid eye movement). Your breathing is timely at this point, your heart rate and blood pressure are that your eyes are jerking rapidly in all directions, and you have your wildest dreams.

In a short period, sleep cycles occur between one-and-a-half to two hours. We spend less time in deep sleep, and more in stages 1, 2, and REM as the cycles increase.

Phase three and four, deep sleep, is the safe cycle where the brain and heart slow down to a rest period, and this phase takes up 50% of sleep time. Dreaming takes place with waking off and on during stage 5. Millions of people suffer from some form of insomnia, leading to tiredness, lack of mental alertness, and physical and mental health weakened. It also leads to accidents involving minor and significant injuries.

Active people are catching fewer colds and infections, but there is no evidence that there is better exercise. It leaves us vulnerable to cold-to-cancer infections, flu-to-heart disease. Several studies found that taking vitamin C (about 600 mg/day) three weeks before an ultra marathon decreased symptoms of a post-race cold, while others found that supplementation with vitamin C did not make any difference. It can be a sign of overtraining or overtaxing your body to get frequent colds. Airborne particles spread cold and flu viruses, so if possible, sneeze into your sleeve or tissue instead of your hands when you cough. You should expect to feel tired and run down when this happens. To be vulnerable to colds and flu and more likely to be infected by infection, germs can easily penetrate the body and cause havoc on your organs if your immune system is not working well.

There are several ways to improve your immune system. Here are some valuable tips for improving the immune system. Immune-strengthening foods involve locally sourced vegetables and fruits, brown bread, beans as well as other legumes, harsh chemicals such as expelled olive oil, hemp oil, walnut oil, flax oil, and butter from coconut. A wealthy citation of selenium, Brazil nuts are especially useful for the immune system. First, antibodies are produced by the immune system that identifies and fend off invaders. The immune system also has integrated memory, it knows how it protected the body against past threats, and it's ready to do it again. Appropriate restful sleep helps heal our bodies and strengthen our minds. Our bodies release strong immune-enhancing substances during deep sleep that enhance immune function.

Everyone has to work instinctively to reset the body clock.

On a median, students go over to bed 1-2hrs later and sleep 1-1,6 hours less than a generation ago. Sleep concerns and depression have increased between many doctors, and college students have realized that it is not necessarily desirable to sleep for nine or more hours a night.

Phase three and four, deep sleep, is the safe cycle where the brain and heart slow down to a rest period, and this phase takes up 50% of sleep time. Dreaming takes place with waking off and on during stage 5. Millions of people suffer from some form of insomnia, leading to tiredness, lack of mental alertness, and physical and mental health weakened. It also leads to accidents involving minor and significant injuries.

Active people are catching fewer colds and infections, but there is no evidence that there is better exercise. It leaves us vulnerable to cold-to-cancer infections, flu-to-heart disease. Several studies found that taking vitamin C (about 600 mg/day) three weeks before an ultra marathon decreased symptoms of a post-race cold, while others found that supplementation with vitamin C did not make any difference. It can be a sign of overtraining or overtaxing your body to get frequent colds. Airborne particles spread cold and flu viruses, so if possible, sneeze into your sleeve or tissue instead of your hands when you cough. You should expect to feel tired and run down when this happens. To be vulnerable to colds and flu and more likely to be infected by infection, germs can easily penetrate the body and wreak havoc on your organs if your immune system is not working well.

There are several ways to boost your immune system. Here are some valuable tips for improving the immune system. Immune-strengthening foods involve locally sourced vegetables and fruits, brown bread, beans as well as other legumes, harsh chemicals such as expelled olive oil, hemp oil, walnut oil, flax oil, and butter from coconut. A wealthy citation of selenium, Brazil nuts are especially useful for the immune system. First, antibodies are produced by the immune system that identifies and fend off invaders. The immune system also has integrated memory, it knows how it protected the body against past threats, and it's ready to do it again. Appropriate restful sleep helps heal our bodies and strengthen our minds. Our bodies release strong immune-enhancing substances during deep sleep that enhance immune function.

Everyone has to work instinctively to reset the body clock.

On a median, students go over to bed 1-2hrs later and sleep 1-1,6 hours less than a generation ago. Sleep concerns and depression have increased between many doctors, and college students have realized that it is not necessarily desirable to sleep for nine or more hours a night.

CHAPTER FIVE

The Effects of Sleep on Muscle Gain

Muscle building requires a lot of concentrated effort and exercise. So because you have to make so much effort for muscle building, you want to make sure that you feed your body correctly and have enough rest, so your exercises pay off. Though, if you don't get enough rest, there are some negative side effects where muscle improvements are concerned. The simple fact is that your muscles grow from the effort you put into your workouts while you sleep. So it's essential to get lots of rest if you want to gain muscle. Your endeavors will not be compensated otherwise.

Recovery Time After spending an hour at the gym and imagining the muscles you build, you must as well be aware that your body needs substantial "return time" from training. Each night is around 8 hours of sleep, and every night, it's not 10 hours tonight and tomorrow for 6 hours because it doesn't work. Your body needs enough sleep every night because the rest is not possible and must be saved every night.

Not all sleep is equal. There are five sleep stages, and if you are like most of the people who live stressful lives, you will never go through stage 1 or 2. That is why you are so exhausted and energy-drained as when you went to bed. If this is the sort of sleep you get, it won't be too beneficial to help you build muscle while you sleep. On the other hand, if you can exercise deep breathing, meditation or other stress relief work before you fall asleep, then you will most likely reach phases 4 and 5 where you can cure, repair and grow. These are the sleep periods that you have to enter if you want to gain muscle. However, given that your body reacts to many different elements in your life, you can not only focus on muscle gain but must also concentrate on stress alleviation, correct eating, and regular exercise.

Deep sleep is essential because the body can repair the muscles torn or broken during the workout during this stage. Also, your body begins the process of special adaptation to imposed demand while you are in a deep sleep. In this process, known as SAID, your body strengthens and strengthens your muscles so that your muscles are prepared once again. This is the method of collecting correct muscles, and if you want to build up muscles, you'll be sure that you not only work outright but also get a lot of deep rest to help the body do its job.

Another advantage, which not many people know, is how your body gets the strength to conduct such tasks in muscle building while you sleep. The reply comes from the fat. That's right, while you are in a deep sleep, and your body works hard to repair and develop your muscles.

So you don't just build up your muscle, you burn fat by merely getting a lot of sleep, which many people won't complain about anyway.

You are now assured that you need to concentrate on having a good night's rest to build muscle, lose weight, and relax the next day.

But, your life is full of family responsibilities, school, work, training, cooking, washing, baking, carpooling and you have not enough hours a day to do everything you need, which will bring you to bed. So, how are you going to get everything you need to do and still sleep for 8 hours each night? The answer is to make it a priority. Your focus should be on your parents, your job, and your rest. You also plan to make your life smoother, so that you can do everything you need to get done and have time to rest. Pay your bills online, for example, and this alone saves you several hours during a month. One idea is if you have to do a lot of washing or go to bed, go to bed and wash tomorrow. It can wait. Prioritizing and understanding that sleep is more important than many things in your life will allow you to relax, develop more muscle, have more energy, and enjoy life.

Muscle building requires a lot of concentrated effort and exercise. So because you have to make so much effort for muscle building, you want to make sure that you feed your body correctly and have enough rest, so your exercises pay off. Though, if you don't get enough rest, there are some negative side effects where muscle improvements are concerned. The simple fact is that your muscles grow from the effort you put into your workouts while you sleep. So it's essential to get lots of rest if you want to gain muscle. Your endeavors will not be compensated otherwise.

Recovery Time After spending an hour at the gym and imagining the muscles you build, you must as well be aware that your body needs substantial "return time" from training. Each night is around 8 hours of sleep, and every night, it's not 10 hours tonight and tomorrow for 6 hours because it doesn't work. Your body needs enough sleep every night because the rest is not possible and must be saved every night.

Not all sleep is equal. There are five sleep stages, and if you are like most of the people who live stressful lives, you will never go through stage 1 or 2. That is why you are so exhausted and energy-drained as when you went to bed. If this is the sort of sleep you get, it won't be too beneficial to help you build muscle while you sleep. On the other hand, if you can exercise deep breathing, meditation or other stress relief work before you fall asleep, then you will most likely reach phases 4 and 5 where you can cure, repair and grow. These are the sleep periods that you have to enter if you want to gain muscle. However, given that your body reacts to many different elements in your life, you can not only focus on muscle gain but must also concentrate on stress alleviation, correct eating, and regular exercise.

What are women in sleep disorders?

Women and sleep problems Evidence is sufficient to show that women are more likely than men to be sleep-related. One of the main reasons is the hormonal makeup of a woman. While hormone levels spike or fall, especially during menstrual cycles, pre- or menopause, and post-pregnancy, women experience more health issues related to sleep than men. Woman is 1.4 times more likely than men to talk about Insomnia. Often, prolonged sleep and sleepiness are sometimes a problem for women.

Sleep disturbances happen to women on a minimal moral basis, but their side effects are abundant. Women have an increased likelihood of stroke or heart disease. Obesity and hypertension are also possible. Because sleep regulates the majority of our body functions, our wellbeing is likely affected by lack of sleep.

Evidence has already shown that youthful women are more likely to sleep than older women. In some instances, women tend to have nap-related problems for their reproductive years. Several factors influence a woman's sleep patterns. Some of them are factors that affect sleep patterns in women. Hormonal changes—hormonal changes in the menstrual cycle can cause sleeplessness or even sleep during the day. In addition to having direct or indirect effects on sleep, moods, and emotions may influence them. This is commonly referred to as premenstrual stress, and nearly 80% of women report it.

Pregnancy–Sleeping patterns can also be affected by pregnancy. Usually, it is noticed that women need more sleep in the first trimester and more during the daytime. These changes and sleep patterns are more comfortable during the second quarter. Many women in the third trimester suffer from sleep loss due to nausea, acidity, excessive urination, cardiovascular, and fetal movements in abnormal periods. Also, lower back pain tends to keep women alert. Sometimes the nasal passage swells, which contribute to sleep apnea and snoring.

Causes related to menstruation and menopause: Menopause and women's aging can cause physical and hormonal changes, causing sleep-related disruptions. There's a propensity to stay awake and anxious during the day. Menopausal woman also suffer from hot flashes and sweats during the night, and this indicates lower levels of estrogen. Deep sleep is not possible at this time and is continuously awake at night.

Insomnia among women Insomnia is the most frequently reported sleep disorder in females, followed by fluctuating sleep patterns, stress, sleepiness during the day, and failure to wake up on time. One of the causes can be mental tension. This is particularly evident in working mothers who tend to ignore exhaustion and other signs that, in the long term, can lead to sleep problems. Insomnia in woman can include the inability to sleep, get deep, or get too early. Many also find it hard to return to sleep when they are awake.

Some of the other gender-specific sleep disorders are Menopausal women with sleep disorders. This leads to loud snoring and deep sleep disturbed. Most women can not go back to sleep and often get tired during the day. This is a time when sleep apnea arises in women over the age of 50 years.

Women also have restless leg syndrome (RLS) or regular limb movement disorder (PLMD). Both of them can be very unsettling to bed. The real reasons for these conditions are not understood. RLS appears to be formed just before a person sleeps, and the calves are continually stressed. The stress can be relieved by movement, which sometimes occurs quite accidentally. PLMD leads to periodic leg movements that tend to awaken somebody. It is also a source of sleeplessness. Sometimes it induces unnecessary sleep, and it has the opposite effect. These two conditions are common in the elderly.

Excessive sleepiness is called narcolepsy during the day. Sleep attacks and so-called cataplexy characterize it. There's an unaccountable desire to sleep when the asleep attack is carried out, while cataplexy is marked by a sudden loss of muscle tonality which contributes to an unjustified emotional episode. There is also often sleep paralysis or hypnagogic hallucinations.

Today, women tend to play multiple roles–workers, daughters, parents, carers, and more. Sleep deprivation is a natural result, often with shortened periods for itself and extreme stress levels. Erratic work and habits often tend to cause sleep problems, which in hormone imbalances are further accentuated.

It is comforting for many women to take some caffeine or nicotine close to bedtime. These are stimulants, however, and often do not help induce sleep. The same goes for vices such as alcohol, which can result in fragmented sleep and nightmares. Sleep disorders are frequently seen in older women.

Overweight places a woman in danger of sleeping problems. Then there are three disorders common to obese women. The symptoms tend to overlap in many cases.

Overweight Inability to fall asleep: This is often seen by younger women who are overweight and is directly related to an unhealthy lifestyle and a very stressed existence.

Inability to sleep: For a variety of reasons, people who are overweight always get excited. The last trimester of pregnancy, chronic arthritis, and the possible intake of pain-related medication may be other health reasons.

Constant sleepiness in the daytime: Most menopausal women are exhausted during the day. Nasal passages sometimes become blocked, and this leads to loud snoring, which also prevents good sleep.

There are several reasons why women struggle when it comes to women and sleep problems. It is the natural order of things in many cases based on a woman's hormonal state. The signs can be recognized, and immediate assistance from a physician will reduce the symptoms. There are several reasons why women struggle when it comes to women and sleep problems. It is the natural order of things in many cases based on a woman's hormonal state. The signs can be recognized, and immediate assistance from a physician will reduce the symptoms.

How to enhance sleep during menopause

Are you a woman near or during the menopause and beginning to notice changes in sleep patterns? You're not alone. You're not alone. According to the National Sleep Foundation, 61% of menopause women report sleep-related problems during cycles of peri-menopausal, menopausal, or post-menopause from early 1940.

You'll find out what the menopausal condition and your sleep have in common, what common treatments you can take to relieve your condition, and what you can do if you still can't sleep after taking these steps.

Our body temperature influences the consistency of our sleep during menopause. The body temperature falls by up to 2-3 degrees during a reasonable sleep period. It helps the brain to cool down and allows us to enter the state of "wintering." Our bodies go into deep sleep here and can work on their restoration and repair work at night, which allows us to get refreshed and alert the next day.

During menopause, your levels of hormones are changing (decreasing estrogen levels), which can give you hot flashes when your body temperature is higher. If this happens during sleep, the regular sleep cycle counters and maintains a higher body temperature than should be necessary to allow restful sleep.

Up to 85% of women have hot flashes for about five years. During hot flashes, the heart rate and peripheral blood circulation usually increase and lead to higher skin temperature, accompanied by suction. As the suddenness evaporates, your body cools down, and you may feel cool. Such events take place at different times of the day for different women, morning, late evening, and bed also called night sweats. Night sweat is the most upsetting because it affects not only our immediate sleep need but also our feeling of well-being the next day. Excessive sleep, irritability, anxiety, and depressed moods can occur during the day due to disturbed sleep.

During menopause Estrogen Replacement Therapy (ERT) or hormonal replacement therapy (HRT) are common medical treatments for menopausal symptoms. Both therapies have been shown to help with menopause symptoms at a cost. Clinical studies have shown that women who undergo such treatments are more likely to suffer from disorders ranging from breast and cardiovascular diseases to dementia.

More recent research has produced both better hormone therapies and alternatives in the field of sleep and topical treatments such as creams. The side effects that come with chemically based treatments have been reduced, but not eliminated.

Parallel attempts have also been made to understand how menopause affects women for the environment and behavior, and the following tips provide an excellent basis to relieve sleep problems while exploring therapeutic choices.

Creating a stimulating atmosphere to sleep: comfortable and supportive mattress, reducing distraction in the bedroom (ideally remove Television, no job, no laptop/computer), great. Adjust your sleeping environment. Use only for sleep and sex, quiet and dark.

Using 45 watt light bulbs in your bedroom: the intense light (100w+) confuses our internal clocks to make us believe it is still dawn, causing us trouble sleeping.

Make a habit of waking up every morning at the same time: it helps to regulate and train our internal clock.

Prevent sleep during the day: napping can disturb sleep at night for people who have sleep problems by increasing their need for sleep regularly.

Make a habit of sleeping every night at the same time: helps to regulate and train our internal timepiece.

Please spend at least two hours per day in sunlight: spending time in the sun helps calibrate the internal time that drives our will to sleep during the night.

Regular exercise—usually late afternoon or early evening: it helps to control our internal clock and metabolism. It increased body temperature and prevented sleep just before going to sleep.

Eat moderately large and healthy meals: and allow for 3-4 hours between dinner and bedtime. It will enable us to complete our digestive system before we go to sleep.

Drink plain yogurt before bedtime: plain yogurt contains low sucre levels, breaks very gradually in your stomach, and does not give rise to sugar while we sleep.

Afternoon avoid caffeine (coffee, caffeine tea, soda, candy, etc.): caffeine stays 7-8 hours in the blood and is a boost that can stop sleep.

Avoid spicy food at dinner: the connections between tasty food and sleep disturbance are known.

Remove nicotine: nicotine is a stimulant and remains there for a long time once in the blood system.

Especially before bedtime, avoid alcohol: alcohol contains sugar that takes 3-4 hours to break down. It helps people wind up and sleep, but wakes them up with a sugar surge in the middle of the night.

Improve your training for mental sleep Practices yoga or meditation regularly (2-3 times a week): these practices help us to master the calming methods needed to make you sleep deep and healthy. If prayer is part of your everyday routine, note it's also a form of relaxation.

Keep a diary of sleep: log on when you go to bed, wake up, and experience interruptions at night. This simple method helps us to understand and measure the complexity of our problem. We will review the data and acknowledge the progress as we make improvements.

Reduce stress and concern: use a worry log to clarify your concerns. It helps to remove troublesome thoughts from your mind to a piece of paper the next day. Sharing your menopause experiences with your friends and family can also reduce stress and concern by putting things in perspective.

Allow 3-4 weeks to follow these easy and simple steps. Make sure you track the progress and sustain the new habits that make a difference. If you find that these changes to your sleeping environment and behavior, and that you still do not sleep profoundly or satisfyingly, it might be time for a sleep coach.

A coach's will: teach how to transcend limiting sleep and menopause assumptions allow you to differentiate between menopause and other past life events and incidents that can influence your sleep, and to build a more healthy way of thinking about trauma and other activities of past life.

Your Sleep Cycle-What are the various stages?

Have you ever stopped to realize that a third of your life is spent sleeping? Yes, sleep takes longer than any other operation every day. But what happens during our sleep?

Many people heard of REM and slept without REM. REM is the time we dream about, or Rapid Eye Movement sleep. The remainder of the period of sleep consists of non-REM sleep.

Non-REM sleep is divided into four fundamental stages. We cycle in these stages all night long, with each cycle culminating in REM sleep. The cycle lasts from 90 to 110 minutes and then repeats.

Our bodies need deep sleep early in the night, which means we spend more of our sleep cycle in the deep-sleep phase. During the night, we relax and spend more time in REM sleep.

To understand the phases of sleep, it is essential to know how scientists measure the cycle of sleep. The first measurement is performed using an electroencephalogram or EEG. The EEG measures the brain waves while you are sleeping. A different brain wave pattern characterizes each phase. The next assessment consists of an electromyogram and an EMG signal of the muscle. This measures the effect of various sleep stages on the muscles. An electrooculogram or EOG mostly calculates the movement of the eyes.

Waking Your brain is quite active when you are awake. Your brain waves have a high frequency, which means they occur close together in a graph with a low amplitude, which means that they are short without any big spikes in a graph. The brain wave deos not follow a regular pattern but change regularly throughout your day. These waves of the brain are known as beta waves.

You become more regular when you relax your brain waves. The amplitude increases, and the frequency slows down. These waves of the brain are called Alpha waves.

Phase 1 When you first go to bed, the first phase of sleep occurs. Enter restful state in which you sleep mostly but still wake quickly. When you float in a semiconscious state, your eyes can move slowly. Sleepers will sometimes experience "sleep starts," where sudden muscle contractions, known as hypnic myoclonic or myoclonic jerks, cause a sense of decrease. When you slumber, the brain waves slow further than you relax, moving into a higher frequency, the more significant wave of amplitude is called the Theta wave. Stage 1 sleep usually doesn't last very long.

Phase 2, is more straightforward than phase 1. Stage 2 Your pupils are no longer moving, and the waves of your brain are slowing. Occasional blasts of fast brain activity known as sleep spindles and times of wavelength called K complexes are characteristic of stage 2 sleep. Some brain waves are stage 2 sleep Theta waves. Like sleep at stage 1, sleep at stage two lasts only a few minutes.

Phase 3 As you sink deeper into the night, the brain falls into a sluggish pattern called the Delta Waves. This is the end of a deep sleep. Your body is relaxed, your eyes still, and you sleep deeply. In stage 3, just under 50% of your brain waves are delta waves with higher peaks between the quieter stages.

Stage 4 This stages are characterized by the activity of the Delta Wave Brain as well as step 3. More than 50% of your brain waves are delta waves, but there are occasionally explosions of higher activity. It's tough to make a person sleep from stage 4. Interestingly, the majority of sleep, night terrors, and even bedwetting are during stage 4 sleep. Stage 4 sleep lasts the best in the early part of the night but slowly falls with the day, until it almost disappears in the morning.

REM After the body cycled from stage 1 to stage 4, it will change its course and return to step 1 before it sleeps in REM. As you start to dream, your body changes a lot. Your breathing is rapid and erratic, your eyes sometimes shift jerky, and your heart rate gets higher. At the same time, your brain waves are involved, much like those, you're waking up to. The body produces a chemical that paralyzes the muscles while you sleep so that you don't thrash or hurt yourself. This is assessed by the EMG, which unexpectedly induces a dramatic muscle tone loss. You'll probably remember the dream in full detail if you're woken during REM sleep.

CHAPTER SIX

No more antidepressants and pills to bed.

Did you know that sleep is so vital to the normal functioning of your body?

You would face most issues without it. Very often, we all have some difficulty sleeping at some stage but for various reasons. Although usual, regular sleep failure can be a sign of a sleep disorder.

If you have some sleep problems such as disturbed sleep, heavy sleep, or complete absence, you should seek some help. These symptoms can seriously affect the strength, health, and emotional stability of your body.

The length of your sleep depends on several factors, but age is the only significant factor. The child's sleep is 10-12 hours, teens about 9 hours, while you should sleep as an adult for at least six hours each day. Many of us are bad sleepers.

The most common sleep disorder is sleeplessness, mostly between women and the elderly. Sleep apnea, snoring, sleep deprivation, and restlessness are also common to sleep issues. Upon proper diagnosis, most of these conditions can be easily managed.

But why is it so important to sleep? As mentioned earlier, your wellbeing and hormones need good sleep to maintain their best. Improves your heart function-Reduces pressure, anxiety, and chronic inflammation-Make your body more healthy and your mind more alert, clearer, and concentrated-Enough sleep will improve your memory-A number of changes in your brain and blood are found when you have good body sleep. Coffee, antidepressants, smoking, or even alcohol can change the patterns of your sleep.

Sleepiness, tiredness, stress, weight gains, impaired thinking capacity, accelerated aging, and lack of concentration are among the most severe cases. This is because the nerves regulate the turning of your brain as you fall asleep.

If you want to learn how to sleep well, you must start by turning off all devices, from a TV, computer, and other home electronics or devices that may disturb your sleep before you go to bed. Dim the lights, take a bath, brush your teeth, pray, meditate in bedtime preparation.

When you go to sleep eventually, relax, stop reading, look at the ceiling, and worry about the issues during the day. This will help you fall into a peaceful sleep and slowly.

Apart from all of these, the sound was discovered to cause the deepest sleep and relaxation. To enter the highest stages of meditation, it takes dedication, patience, and discipline. However, some soothing music can help you relax your mind better and reach the highest meditation levels.

The human brain cells continue to move rhythmically with certain specific sound frequencies, according to scientific research. Audio brainwaves go a long way to harness the power of the mind and drive the brain to sleep in peace.

The audio brainwave is more comfortable as you can easily pack the device in your bag when traveling to minimize undesired noise, such as on the train, airplane, or bus. You will never find difficulty falling or sleeping with outstanding audio quality.

A healthy, safe, and properly regulated nervous system produces appropriate brain waves at the appropriate levels in a given situation and promptly. It explains how auditory brain waves are much more powerful than any other treatment currently on the market as a sound therapy or medication for sleeping problems.

The experimental application of multifaceted sound stimulation has been demonstrated to elicit the desired state of mind, from relaxation to depths of sleep and meditation. Pure tones from the natural world work perfectly well to adjust brainwave patterns.

Studies show that electrical brain stimulation at frequencies between 0.5 and 2 Hz can induce profound relaxation and calmness. In comparison with popular music, ambient or background music is used because it has no recognizable melody parse (there is melody present, but the listener is not identifiable).

A melody familiar or word-laden may confuse the listener because the brain naturally tries to follow a well-known tune or to attend the sung or the spoken word, which interferes with brainwave learning and the desired effect.

Are you conscious that your speech and language centers are in the left hemisphere of the brain?

This area may thus become tired or distracted after a tiring day or long period of activity, and it explains why your attention and focus might seem distracted after a busy day. To solve your sleep problem with the best results, stereo headphones are recommended but are not necessarily necessary because they cancel any noise that distracts your focus. The use of a music visualizer, such as those for computer applications, will improve the experience better.

The condition of your brainwave affects virtually every aspect of your life's experiences. For example, if you have trouble concentrating or even sleep, it means that you are in the wrong brainwave state when it comes to contesting what you want to do.

No need to worry, as with this plan, you can monitor your mental condition to achieve whatever mental condition you need. Feel calm, happy, imaginative, and concentrated on making your dreams come true in audio brainwave life.

The audio frequencies are so powerful in bringing you into a relaxed relaxation state that will lead to profound changes in your everyday life. You can also choose your taste music whenever you want.

It works by using unique tones and pulses to influence the patterns of your brain waves, by soothing music that leads to deep sleep. This technology is unbelievably powerful, wholly secure and improves what your brain does naturally, and brings you to deep sleep in minutes.

If you hit the PLAY button while you're sleeping, the end of the recording is probably never heard with or without headphones.

Tell yourself goodbye to sleep problems and insomnia and wake up in a pleasing mood for a refreshing morning.

The technology of audio brainwave is the future, and the brain can produce balanced, positive, and curative brainwaves while you continue to use it. No coffee, antidepressants, or sleeping pills are required. Act intelligently, but use this incredible technology to achieve deep and stable states of consciousness. You only have to press the button to unleash your power to read, meditate, focus, recover, and sleep.

Take control of life and mind. You can avoid your sleeplessness by having the natural sleep cure, the audio brainwave, the learning recording designed to keep you in a deep, safe and restorative state of sleep. Use the science of your rhythms to fix electric imbalances that keep you alert and make you feel relaxed and normal.

Develop an overnight routine to help your baby sleep

Most babies wake up when they're tired, irritated, and breathing obstructed at the end of a sleep cycle. Research suggests that waking up during sleep cycles is a critical mechanism for survival. If the sleep state of the baby was so high that it could not express its needs, its well-being could be compromised. Families should, therefore, not feel under pressure to sleep their newborn baby too long, too deeply, too early. A sleeping pattern usually begins between 3 and 6 months old, and a child may sleep for five or more hours.

The two major problems for most parents are getting their baby to sleep and to sleep. Many babies sleep quickly and sleep while others sleep comfortably, but wake up sometimes. Many babies have difficulty sleeping, but stay sleeping while others don't want to go to bed or eat. Sleeping problems can arise when babies are high sleepers six months old and vice versa. There are many reasons why babies have trouble sleeping, but knowing about the different phases and what to do when the baby wakes up in the night can be helpful.

Babies experience five sleep cycles, each lasting approximately one hour. We spend twice the amount of time sleeping and productive than sleeping. The baby's muscles relax, and her eyelids flutter during the first phase of light sleep. She can twitch, cough, suck, and breathe irregularly. When a child is put in her cot, she will wake up. The baby's extremities relax during deep sleep, and her hands open, and breathing is relaxed and standard. Baby enters the frenzied period of active sleep after a deep sleep. During this point, they grimace and panic, tense and jerk the muscles accidentally, dabbing the eyes in all directions and rapid breathing and heart rate. The time between the end of restless sleep and the next sleep cycle is the most vulnerable.

Many babies whimper and wake up after a period of sleep. However, they may drift back to sleep if they are not disturbed. If your baby needs to be fed or a change, keep it as low as possible and put it in its crib or cot when it meets your needs. Do not pick her up, talk to her, make eye contact, play the music, or communicate with her in any way, or she will demand the same treatment if she wakes up, when her baby is not hungry or upset. Just put your hand on your child to console it, until it falls asleep again. After a few days, she gets used to the new routine and sleeps by herself still. When you pay too much attention to your infant, waking and playing at irregular times may be extended into late childhood.

Bedtime routine One thing the sleep experts agree is that a regular bedtime routine, predictable, consistent is necessary. It does not matter what the routine is to do the same every night. The baby will soon learn to associate such activities and circumstances with bedtime, while new sleep patterns may take her a week or two. After a routine is established, stick to it every night consistently.

These are some tips that can help: o Let your baby take a good kick to pull out.

o If your baby gets out, helps to relax in a warm bath, the more relaxed environment will lower its temperature and trigger the sleep mechanism.

O Massage your baby or read a story to help her relax.

o Into unique clothing that is used only at bedtime, put your baby.

O Swaddle your baby in a blanket of cotton or put it in a cot sleeping bag to remind her of the womb's warmth and comfort.

o Use phrases such as' Bed Time' and' Night Night' to help your baby sleep.

o After you wind and sleep your baby, otherwise she might be surprised to find that when she wakes, you do not have your comforting arms.

o Make a regular habit of sleeping in a crib or cot.

o Ensure that the room is dark and silent. It helps to differentiate between night and day.

Everyone has a latency in sleep before going to sleep, so don't wait until the baby sleeps in her cot. For most children, crying for no genie reason before sleep is also common. Sometimes, after a busy day, your baby has to relax, and cry makes her sleepy.

Ways of Using White Noise For Better Sleep

Were you aware that we spend a third of our lives sleeping? It is therefore of great advantage that your bedroom and sleeping environment is relaxing, calming, and relaxing for good quality sleep.

Find your room cool, calm, and comfortable. Use darkening blinds or curtains to block light and play soothing white noise to lock noise and create a soothing sleeping atmosphere). The aim is to ensure 7 to 8 hours of quality restful sleep to maintain good health and long and productive life.

Were you aware that we spend a third of our lives sleeping? It is therefore of great advantage that your bedroom and sleeping environment is relaxing, calming, and relaxing for good quality sleep.

Find your room cool, calm, and comfortable. Use darkening blinds or curtains to block light and play soothing white noise to lock noise and create a soothing sleeping atmosphere). The aim is to ensure 7 to 8 hours of quality restful sleep to maintain good health and long and productive life.

8. Please spend some time outside in the sun. Daylight exposure will help you to sleep better.

Tips for bedtime 1. The only ones whose bodies react well to a sleep schedule are babies and children. Try to keep your sleep and wake up regularly. Try to keep the routine on holidays and days off if necessary. Going to bed at the same time will put your body into a healthy habit every night.

2. Have a daily bedtime "routine," like a hot shower or ample tub, accompanied by reading or listening to music. Extension, yoga, and meditation can also be of great help. If you do these rituals regularly each night, your body is told that the time to sleep is close.

3. Some deep, slow breathing can help to relax. Take your nose slow deep breaths, and you'll see your belly expand. Then exhale all your pressure out of your body slowly. Experience the pressure with every emits from your body. Do 10 of these deep, slow breaths to get rid of stress and relax when preparing for a beautiful night of good sleep.

4. Make sure you have a quiet, dark, and comfortable bedroom. Sound and light can interfere with your sleep ability

5. Just use the bed for sleep and sex. Remove distraction items such as reading materials, laptops, and TVs for work and study. Watching the news in bed at night with death, violence, war, and destruction stories can be too stimulating and decrease your sleeping capacity.

6. Lots people find it easier to sleep in the bed with an electric fan. It's great until the cold autumn and winter come when you don't want to blow a cold wind. To enjoy the soothing and relaxing fan sound, search for a fan cd with a white noise sound to maximize efficiency.

7. Aromatherapy can also be useful at bedtime. The soothing fragrances like Vanilla and Lavender can be very calming and relaxing. But don't leave your sleeping candle burning! You could enjoy the new scented, much safer scabbard diffusers than candles.

8. Stop living with pets. Animals can interfere with quality sleep.

9. If you can not sleep, get out of bed and watch TV, browse the internet, read, or anything else that can help you to relax. Then come back to your bed when you are ready again to sleep.

I hope that in your quest for relaxation, sleep, and sleep, these sleep tips are useful and helpful. Good sleep aims to wake up and revitalize you, ready to face your day.

How to deal with elderly sleeping conditions

When an older man had a late-night snack, his grandmother often saw him sitting on favorite chair of her sewing until late at night. I recall telling her why she was so late and her response, "Now that he was old, it's hard to get your kids to sleep so quickly." She was awoken and good for me because she used to tell me the best stories late at night.

Sleeping disorders are indeed the most common problems affecting the elderly today. You may have trouble sleeping or waking up in the middle of the night and then find it hard to go back to sleep and sleep.

Nonetheless, the amount of nightly sleep we have to sleep in old age is the same as we wanted when we were younger. The various diseases and medications were found to be responsible for today's sleep disorders among the elderly.

Aging also affects the rhythm of the circadian body or the natural clock that can change the time of sleep. That's why your mom sleeps early at 10 and gets up to 4 doing yoga. Specific factors affecting the clock of the body include lack of physical activity, a lack of mental stimulation, and an early bedtime.

Insomnia or sleep deprivation and narcolepsy or excessive sleep are types of sleep disorders.

Sleeplessness or insomnia affects nearly half of adults aged 60 and over. Insomnia may be caused by an underlying medical condition or by a side effect of a medication called secondary insomnia in some cases. It is known as primary insomnia in the absence of a causative factor. Women tend to complain about insomnia more than men; it may be due to the period after menopause.

Narcolepsy is a neurological condition that causes intense sleepiness, and can even cause someone to sleep unexpectedly and without warning. There are no known direct causes of narcolepsy, but there is a lack of hypocretin, a brain chemical that controls sleep and waking. Even after sleep at night, "wake assaults" by people with narcolepsy make it harder for people to live healthy lives.

Causes of sleep disturbance: Chronic pain: the various pains in the back of the legs come with age. For some, this pain could prevent them from sleeping. Even when sleeping, the body keeps registering pain. The body is deprived of the growth hormone released during deep sleep, which assists a body healing mechanism with constant pain and light sleep. With no rest, the feeling of pain always rises the next day, so it continues as an infinite loop.

Apnea Sleep: Obstructive sleep apnea (OSA) is more common in older adults, affecting about 40% of adults. In this case, the upper airway gets too small by relaxing the windpipe muscles. Those who have sleep apnea often stop breathing in a single night, usually for one minute or longer or hundreds of times.

The choices are to stop alcohol and muscle relaxants or weight loss, but other remedies do not work, sleep on the foot, sleep 30 degrees high, and use CPAP maskings.

Restless Limb Syndrome: this condition causes pain in the arms, such as pins and needles. Periodical motions in the limbs make people jump and kick their legs in sleep every 20 to 40 seconds. One study found that nearly 35 percent of older adults have this disorder at least mildly.

Lack of rest Limb Syndrome can cause chronic insomnia and one of the factors contributing to everyday fatigue. Many solutions include folic acid and iron supplements, pre-sleeping runs, and mindfulness relaxation techniques.

Urinary problem: Elderly people often wake up to urinate many times in the night. This is known as nocturia. Because of their age, the body decreases the production of anti-diuretic hormone, which slows down urine output and prefers to have full blood at night. Also, with age, the size of the bladder decreases and, therefore, frequently visits the washroom.

Solutions reduce fluids before sleep, not diuretics such as alcohol.

Depression, stress, and worries: Most elderly people are worried and have a negative effect on their sleeping patterns. When we age, Cortisol raises our susceptibility to stress hormone. This can result in the prevalence of insomnia becoming responsive to these stress hormones.

Even anxiety affects sleep, including stress. People with depression would likely not be satisfied with the amount of sleep they get. Otherwise, not getting enough sleep will also cause depression-like symptoms. For older people, risk factors of depression include spousal loss, disability, social isolation, and the onset of dementia.

Depression can only be combated by taking constructive and optimistic action. Going out, socializing, joining a club are some ways of being optimistic and battling sleep problems.

Medication: Some widely used medicines can stimulate and disrupt sleep. Several antidepressants, decongestants, bronchodilators, anti-hypertensives, and corticosteroids are included among these. Diuretics may cause frequent sleep interruptions at night to go to the bathroom.

Lack of sleep causes: The overall health of the elderly is affected significantly. Research from North Carolina State University indicates that poor sleep is one of the main causes of elderly memory problems.

Functions such as the ability to learn and retain information, coordinate, prepare, and solve problems are also impaired, and attention to concentrate, sustain, and change is affected.

Research shows that sleep is essential to the healing and well-being of illnesses. When patients do not sleep well, they tend to complain more about arthritic pain.

Will you take medicine?

The last way to sleep should be through drugs, as they also have their side effects and can lead to addiction. It is recommended that sleeping pills should not be taken more than two consecutive days and not more than three times a week.

Ways to address it: Below are some of the alternative ways of dealing with sleeping disorders.

Avoid napping, especially after 3 pm during the day.

Don't use the bed for any other activity, but sleep or intimate* Keep your bedroom dark, cool, relaxing, and a little cool* Make your sleep ritual like-having a warm bath, drinking milk, ole massage, before sleeping* if you can't sleep within a 20 minute period in the bed, leave the room and perform some other activity.* Do not take coffee or tea before going to bed* Go back once you're mentally and physically tired Research shows that people with advice about their approach to sleeping have the best long-term chance of a good night's rest than people taking medicine.

Being Old - Or Pretending

We're old when we get to 70 years. In our eighties, most of us die. We cheat the odds when we reach 90. When we get as old as 100, we have successfully put our finger to destiny... So long as Life continues to last, at least. Our only regret is that our grandkids maybe 120. This didn't happen to us in time... When we watch young people have it better, our usual lamentation is.

The benefits of being old are high, such as the vast experience, much better judgment than most, the productivity of a pro, and a concentration on someone who has stripped his Life to what is necessary.

The latter, most robust of the old virtues, is seen as proof of senility that does not know who we think they should be, a lack for important details leading to acts of self-discussion-which an older adult finds unimportant. This intense, narrow focus of the former is like an absolute inflexibility. Nevertheless, such a narrow perspective is expected from deep expertise and wisdom. By being so well-formed, the microcosm of a highly focused person's Life became a macrocosmic model. Anywhere applicable.

On the other hand, there are some terrible aspects, such as chronic and never-ending illness. You have to become used to pain that doesn't end. You need to adapt to the pain and care for yourself better. Yeah, you should take medicine because you know that Life hurts. But there's still pain. Even extreme drugs give up Life before they are done.

This does not mean that you can sometimes not do anything about aging illness, especially when you walk as much as you can every day. Don't hesitate for stuffed or wheelchairs, no matter how superbly convenient and smartly mechanical they are—no matter how much hurt you're going to get forced to. Stop walking, and our body dies more quickly. It needs to be encouraged to remain alive... Healthy, what could be considered prodding by some. Exercise becomes more important, not less important as we get older. If we also pay close attention to your body, it will reveal that a lot of sorrow is caused by our poor sitting habits, which chair, where, how, how and what pillows and blankets we sleep, how we relax, how we steep and raise our shoulders unconsciously and all the time in response to tension or unknown fear, etc. A typical example: hands hanging on top of the head cause very painful problems in the old age, which involve aspirin every four hours.

The big downside of the old one is that Life is almost over. To think all the time and effort we put into Life, including everything we have learned, ironed out, it's a piece of cake to handle most things. To imagine that experience and skill die in just one moment, then suddenly, we are only a smoke pot that quickly dissipates into nothing. The final blow is worse than any other period of a letdown. What once was there, full of life, is gone forever, out of reach. Yeah, many people recall, even dreadfully miss us. This isn't our Life, however. In that, we have only become part of the Life of someone else... Their memory. Their memory. How much they love us doesn't matter. We're no longer there.

Most young people fear death, so they make up many stories that deny death is going to happen. Whoever is old, and also wise, knows that fear is Life, not death. Death is the time it's just over. Fear is a sign that we are alive. So what are we afraid of? The reply is... Are we going to have regrets? Have we lived our entire life? Are we or were we doing anything meaningful?

The answer is always, and maybe it will always be no! Most of our lives and skills are wasted for someone else's sake. It took us most of our Life to find out what we could have been with little time to do anything about it. Even in democracies, today, lives are not established to give the evolution and the enlightenment of individual people the most excellent support. The primary direction of Life is still cultural, not private. Life is designed to program us all to give our lives to a social purpose, first and foremost, if we were someone who wanted to change social goals.

Death is so frightening that most of us pretend that it never happens. This scares us, thus, and surprises us. We're shunning it. In so doing, we avoid the hardest lesson that people will ever have to learn, which is that Life is as negative as it is positive. Avoid the negative, to stay always in the positive, and happiness becomes a shame. Only such a robust pretense would make money the essential thing in human life as if it could gain something actual. Death and our fear of its negative consequences reveal how vacant and inhuman a company is.

CHAPTER SEVEN

The connection Between
Diabetes and Apnea Sleep

Moreover, an additional reason for losing weight overweight can not only increase the likelihood of a person developing obstructive sleep apnea, but also the probability of developing type 2 diabetes — excess fat around the stomach and intestines of a sleeper press and blocks the airways. A deafening noise is generated when the air is cut off, which often wakes the sleeper. This causes highly disturbed sleep, which can lead to reduced levels of activity, which can exacerbate type 2 diabetes. Even if a person is not fully awakened, there have been frequent interruptions of the oxygen flow.

OSA is not just painful for the patient but also painful for anyone who has to live with the patient. In contrast to most snoring, OSA's volume is noted. The unexpected gagging and shaking sounds that the producer can not wake up would undoubtedly wake up any visitors to your house or your girlfriend. Some OSA patients are so loud that in every room of a home, they can be heard. It stigmatizes OSA patients, including families and friends, who can dissuade a patient from even losing weight. Yet obesity is an even worse choice.

Results of a major Canadian study reported in the October 2009 issue of' Thorax' that, although the ideal weight of your body was preserved, OSA sleepiness led to the development of type 2 diabetes. OSA doubled and tripled the risk of developing type 2 diabetes among study participants. More than 2,100 Canadian men and women have voluntarily participated in the OSA study. A volunteer's average age was 50, about ten years before type 2 diabetes. This suggests that even people with OSA must take careful account of their diet and exercise practices.

The good news is that diabetics can not only better manage their blood sugar level by losing weight but can also lead to a significant drop in OSA noise. This is a result of a Random study of the effect of weight loss on obese patients with diabetes Type 2 obstructive sleep apnea. As part of their diabetes management, the category of weight loss was the strongest, with some losing all traces of OSA. Many volunteers are over 60 years of age, at a time when overweight people are most at risk for diabetes.

The authors of the study suggest that overweight, diabetic patients require medical or psychological intervention not just to advise them on how to achieve weight loss objectives, but also to ensure that they achieve the objectives. When a person with diabetes loses weight, they must gain enough energy to keep exercising regularly.

What is obstructive apnea for sleep?

This does not mean that weight loss will help all forms of sleep apnea, just OSA. Sleep apnea may also be caused by throat or soft palate deformation or growth. This mass or deformity causes the sudden blockage of the airways of the sleeper. In such cases, apnea can only be eliminated by surgery in the affected areas.

But OSA differs because the airways of the sleeper are blocked by external airway pressure. During deep sleep, the muscles of the body relax. This usually leads to a sleeper's mouth being open at night. The remaining open-jaw movement can cause sufficient pressure to create the complete blockage of the airway. If the apnea is mild, sleep aids like the dental mouthpiece will often be used to prevent the opening of the mouth during deep sleep.

Yet counter medicines and dental aids do not support severe OSA patients whose airways can be blocked by up to 30 an hour. These patients are often asked to use an oxygen machine for continuously positive airway pressure (CPAP). The patients must then attempt to sleep with a face mask to prevent blockages of airways. Many OSA patients dislike the CPAP system, not really. If you are overweight, you can only get a good night's sleep by getting a stringent weight loss program to avoid your progress to Type 2 diabetes.

What about the Surgery of Bariatrics?

The bariatric procedure, also known as gastric bypass surgery, is a very vigorous choice for weight loss. Although this severe form of weight loss can temporarily alleviate symptoms of type 2 diabetes and sleep apnea, patients frequently regain weight unless a patient maintains diet and exercise. You also may have OSA-related problems or see such complications just months after surgery.

Bariatric surgery does not decrease OSA, as well. Bariatric surgery advocates claim that studies on OSA patients were too small to be accurate. Recent American veterans at Walter Reed Memorial Hospital show only a 4 percent reduction in airway shutdowns in 24 patients who had surgery one year after the procedure. There seemed to be immediate benefits, but after one year, most of them vanished. The OSA conclusion is a painful and embarrassing problem that reduces the quality of life. It increases the chance for the individual to become a diabetic type 2.(' Obstructive Sleep Apnea After Surgical Weight Loss '; CJ Lettieri et al.;' The Journal of Clinical Sleep Medicine'; 2008.) The problem is compounded by being overweight. There are no shortcuts for weight loss management of OSA and type 2 diabetes. The bariatric activity does not offer significant long-term benefits. OSA can only be controlled successfully by careful diet and weight loss.

New Age Dawning - Sleep Well, Breathe Well

,Early to rise means you have early go to bed, makes a man healthful, wealthy and wise." This brief proverb can be traced as far back as 1496, and even earlier, if you take all of its variants into account. People seem to have always recognized the need for a good night's sleep, but quality sleep today has become a privilege, not a requirement. Yet sleepless walking may not be so easy because your body can not easily do without it.

"More people sleep less than 6 hours a night, and sleep difficulties confuse 75 percent of ourselves at least a few nights a week," according to a recent Harvard Health Publications survey. "Most people are inadequately sleeping and, as a result, chronic fatigue poses a significant problem for millions of Americans.

But there's still those who are tired and uncomfortable with the "catch up" sleep on the weekends, no matter how much sleep they get. In such circumstances, there is something else that may be awkward: the patients feel that sleepiness is usually the result and not the actual cause. It could be their poor night breathing and not the amount of sleep they are deprived of.

Whenever you are trained in a certain way, you almost always have to take long, deep breaths and concentrate on your breathing. The control of your breath, especially as it relates to your stamina and endurance, from Pilates to yoga to running and Tai Chi, is critical to maintaining good shape and gaining control.

But consider what if you couldn't breathe well while you were sleeping. You would get more than a body flabby. You would have been headed for some serious health problems. But it's precisely what happens if you suffer from obstructive sleep apnea or OSA in short.

Have breathing difficulties while sleeping?

While all people have different levels of airway narrowing, people with sleep apnea or its milder variant UAS have more likely anatomies to break down than others. If you have a facial triangular shape, a long neck, a comprehensive, stuck neck such as a football player, or if you have a higher tongue in your arches (see diagram), all of these anatomical factors can prevent you from getting airways obstructed or having respiratory problems while you are sleeping. Obesity and weight is not the primary indicator of sleep apnea as it was once assumed.

For some patients with OSA or UARS, sleeping on their sides and their stomachs is a necessary condition in getting a good night's rest. That position gives the tissue around the airway a bit longer flexibility than sleeping on their backs, and their tongues appear to collapse not so quickly if they are lying flat on their back, in general during deep sleep when the throat muscles are more relaxed.

Although many UARS and OSA patients think they prefer to sleep this way just because they always slept like this, for a good reason, they may have chosen to sleep like this. It's almost like a reflective survival mechanism since these preferences to sleep on our sides and stomachs could not be formed through a conscious effort but as a mechanism for reflective coping with something that is distressing us. That is why when patients come to me with sinuses and or chronic fatigue problems, I always ask,' Who do you like to sleep in?' It's almost exact if patients want to sleep on their sides or stomachs, when I look at their airway with my video endoscopes, that their airways will look like a coffee stirrer opening.

Although many of us understand intuitively that breathing is necessary for life, those who have sleep apnea or UARS don't breathe for life. Although they sleep and therefore have time to reset and replenish their brain, muscles and organs, apnea, and frequent breathing cessation interrupt this process regularly. It is like your "fight or flight" response is continually going on, although it takes time off. Think about your car if the ignition is never switched off. Okay, this is what happens to patients with sleep apnea.

Sleep Apnea Issues It has many serious consequences, many of which can be avoided, but, as I mentioned earlier because so many people who have this disorder are unconscious.

Research has shown, for one thing, that sleep apnea has a higher incidence of high blood pressure and cardiac disease. Many patients who have already received high blood pressure medication or a history of heart disease are found to have some respiratory sleep disorder.

Diabetes, depression, and numerous anxiety problems are some other chronic conditions related to sleep apnea. Many of the exhaustion and attention deficit disorders, such as ADHD, have also been associated with sleep apnea in children. A recent study discover that a high percentage of children who undergo tonsillectomy with clear OSA symptoms showed a significant change in their ability to focus and pay attention in schools, if not a substantial reduction in their behavior problems. As you see, respiring poorly as you sleep can have severe implications for both the elderly and the young.

Because sleeping well is almost synonymous with feeling good, looking young and healthy to people, most people disregard their breathing as an essential matter of life. We don't know that this is where life comes from.

People don't often say, "How well I breathed last night," if in the morning they feel tired and hesitant. Some people then focus on the amount of sleep they have or don't have. This may be why in America today, sleep pills and anti-anxiety drugs are so popular.

However, as everybody jumps on the new anti-aging rage, the breathing in the medical community is not becoming a secondary but a tertiary issue. Breath is often a matter of fact in the framework of holistic and preventive medicine. Though many proponents of these therapies also breathe as the way to reduce stress and enhance mental well-being they often neglect this when providing nutritional and herbal supplements such as sleep aids with little or no consideration for the fact that none of these regiments are all that effective unless there is an effective mechanism for sleep. It's almost like an automotive owner shooting premium petrol with vehicles with broken fuel lodges for customers. Earlier or later, this car will either break down or stop dead in its tracks, or at least waste the first thing you put in to make it work better. Furthermore, no pills or supplements, regardless of how potent, can effectively fix your sleep problems if your sleep problems originate in an anatomical problem, such as your airway. These issues must be addressed from the source of the airway.

Bottles of air to OSA and UARS patients, you could take simple measures to improve your breathing while you sleep if you suspect it can be the cause of your problems.

The first thing I prescribe to all my patients with exhaustion issues is not to lie on their backs. That is one of the many reasons why snoring often stops when people sleep. The next best thing to do is to shed excess weight if you can not change your sleep position this way due to an injury or habit. However, if you are still tired or have difficulty keeping the focus on work, my recommendation is to take a formal study of sleep or polysomnography to determine the root cause of your day tiredness or exhaustion.

Where do you want me to sleep?

A standard sleep test is conducted in a sleeping laboratory where a sleep technician will put you on a monitor during your sleep, and a so-called "sleep doctor uses the measurements." Though you might or might not be diagnosed officially with OSA even after the sleep study, I have seen many, if not a large majority of these patients obtain valuable information to solve any other sleep problems. Nonetheless, most, if not all, patients who I believe have these conditions have a mild to moderate breathing component that accompany their sleep problems. And for these people, not many sleeping pills target airway obstruction at the root of their sleep problems rather than the underlying respiratory problem.

To understand how important it is to sleep, it's equally important if it's not more important to know how you can get the restorative sleep that you need.

Essentially, sound sleep provides your body with vital services. After a full day learning new skills and new experiences, sleep enables the brain to shut down its mode of learning, absorb and recapture the further information. Adequate sleep also allows the body to produce the correct hormonal balance to help stabilize weight and effectively use carbohydrates (hence, studies show that insufficient sleep is often related to increased weight gain). Sleep sufficiently helps to ensure your health by making your brain more alert and optimized to prevent injury and keep you comfortable and well-adjusted.

Sleep also helps to maintain your body healthy by enhancing your immune function, reducing the chance of certain cancers, and decreasing your blood pressure. In short, you lose one of the most important ways to keep you young and healthy for a long time when you don't sleep well.

But it can be more critical to ensure that your good night sleep is not damaged by breathing problems such as obstructing sleep apnea than that additional hour of a shut-eye. As the new-age old gurus tell us, it's not as early as you are genetical. It's not how old. Also, if your breathing is impaired while you sleep, your health doesn't depend lots on how much you sleep nightly, but how well you sleep in the night, and how well you breathe while sleeping. Briefly, look more closely at what is happening inside and not outside for solutions to your sleep problems. What you find may surprise you.

How to Help a Baby to Sleep

1. Nights without sleep?

Sleep is among the common issues for parents with young children. One thing I'm pleased to kiss as my kids get older is the nights without sleep. Approximately 40 percent of children sleep, which their parents perceive to be problematic.

Sleep is an opportunity for your body and mind to rest and regenerate, to refresh your baby. Deep sleep is the time your child generates the highest growth hormone concentrations. Therefore, this time is essential for the growth of your son. Recent research has also linked sleep deficiency in children under 16 years of age to obesity.

Sleep deprivation can consistently lead to fatigue, irritability, poor memory and concentration, aggression, and depression (in the child and family!).

Nevertheless, it is essential to remember that every child has its unique requirement and that you might have a child who only requires very little sleep. It can be a daunting advantage in later life, as this may be to your sleep (many world leaders get up at 3 am, I am told). Sleep is among the common issues for parents with young children. One thing I'm pleased to kiss as my kids get older is the nights without sleep. Approximately 40 percent of children sleep, which their parents perceive to be problematic.

Sleep is an opportunity for your body and mind to rest and regenerate, to refresh your baby. Deep sleep is the time your child generates the highest growth hormone concentrations. Therefore, this time is essential for the growth of your son. Recent research has also linked sleep deficiency in children under 16 years of age to obesity.

Sleep deprivation can consistently lead to fatigue, irritability, poor memory and concentration, aggression, and depression (in the child and family!).

2. What is my child's average amount of sleep?

You can sleep for about 16 hours a day, waking both day and night, from birth to 6 months. Babies of this age have tiny tummies and must, therefore, feed small and often. It is normal at this stage that there is no distinction between day and night. Smaller babies may need to eat more often, while bigger babies may have to go between feeds for longer.

After six weeks, your baby will be able to go between feeds for more extended periods, and you will notice that the day and night routines start.

Once your baby starts to wean six months, he or she will feel satisfied for a more extended period and can start sleeping for 6 hours plus one to two days at night.

At one year of age, most kids will have lunch day, and by three years, most kids won't have to sleep during the day.

It may be uncommon for your child if you don't stick to this pattern. Another close family members are worth looking at because your child may have inherited his sleep pattern.

3. What can I do to sleep my child well?

A good and consistent bedtime routine is an essential habit. You find something that suits you and your friends, but here are some helpful signs to make other people feel comfortable sleeping with their babies.

4. Take the time to put your child on bed consistently Brush your child's teeth after their bottle and before sleep Bottle of milk or banana before bed can help sleeping (they both contain tryptophan, a substance that helps to induce slept), Brush your baby's teeth after bottle and before sleep. If you wake up during the night, calm him and leave quickly and gently. Finally, your child should be able to sleep alone without your presence.

If a nappy need to change, change it at the very least and then bring it gently back down.

5. Give your child fizzy drinks/caffeine/ candy / flavored sweets in the 2 hours before bed (can contain stimulants) Only allow your child to watch TV or use the computer right before bed When your child wakes at night don't turn on / play with it.

Your child should not need a bottle of milk at night after six months. Stick to bottled water if you think your child might be thirsty.

Don't let a boy cry uncomfortably. Verify that they are not uncomfortable/hurt, then calm them down and leave.

Do not use a bed or bathroom as a penalty 6. Was my child supposed to sleep in his bed?

There are no answers, right or wrong; you must decide what is best for you. Here are some advantages and disadvantages to help make your mind sleep in your bed.

Pros: Your child has its bedroom and doesn't get disrupted by you Your child does not depend on you to sleep at night and again, when he wakes during the night You don't get distracted by your child's noise/wriggling There is no danger of crushing your baby (especially when you drink heavily or take sedation drugs). Are there other tips to sleep, my child?

It is essential to make sure your child does not wake for a reason. Is the room too warm or too cold? Is there a TV or radio in the vicinity? If your baby weeps, snores, itches, or coughes, speak to your GP as they can.

With younger children/infants, it is OK to leave them in their cot if they do not sleep at once.

If you still find it challenging to get your child to sleep, speak to your health visitor and your doctor about sleep training. You may have a health visitor who is a specialist in sleep problems in your area.

If your kid has difficulties in getting to sleep, you can try to snack their day and make sure that they have some physical play during the day (the physical activity recommended for children is one hour every day). Getting out increases your body's amount of melatonin (a hormone sleep promotion), so try to get your child to play out for some time each day.

8. My baby wakes up too soon, what can I do?

Your child may be distracted by sunlight, especially in the summer. Thick blinds or blackout curtains are an ideal way to block the light from the bedroom of your son.

Naturally, most kids are early risers. Make sure you have safe soft toys in your bed or cot if you wake too early. There are sure specialty clocks on the market that can warn your child if it is acceptable to make noise. My daughter had a watch on a rabbit's face, and the rabbit's ears would go up at 6:30 am.

Hang in there. Hang in there. They are usually exhausted and sleep longer when your child begins school.

9. Nightmares and night terrors The child may have nightmares for about two years. A sleepwalk is a vivid lousy dream. Your child may wake up and find it difficult to sleep again. However, nightmares may begin after a traumatic occurrence in your child's life, so this is important for exploring whether your child suddenly begins to have them.

You should ease and reassure them if your child has a nightmare.

Night terrors are different than nightmares because your child may have eyes open but still sleep. You may be distressed or weeping, and this may be upset to watch as a parent, but it won't hurt your child, and you'll see that in the morning, they don't remember the terror.

If your child has a dreadful night, do not wake them, but calm them down and then sleep when you can.

Most children grow up by ten years of age out of both nightmares and night terrors.

10. A child is going to bed, what can we do?

Slumbering is like a nightmare at night because your baby is still sleeping, but instead of being scared or upset, they walk around and speak instead sometimes.

You don't have to wake your baby, lead them back to bed. It is essential to ensure that your child is safe. A stairway through your door can be helpful. Ensure doors and windows are locked, fires are guarded, and knives and instruments are put away.

The Sleeping Disorder Troubles In Insomnia

Good and uninterrupted sleep can be great for everyone every day. But around one in 3 people worldwide are confirmed to be sleeping insomnia. Insomnia was the problem of falling asleep, that was common health problem. This problem occurs mainly with the age of old age, and women are more affected than men. Insomnia may be due to its medical condition or as a sign of other diseases. A person who has it cannot sleep or wake up often during sleep. Insomnia may be short-term insomnia, which lasts a few days or weeks and may be called acute insomnia, or long-term insomnia.

Based on the duration and severity of insomnia, transient insomnia can be classified into three types, temporary insomnia caused by journeys, relocation, or by certain external factors such as light, sound, etc. that curbs healthy sleep. It could last for one or two nights.

Short term insomnia: insomnia of this kind can last several weeks, mainly caused by mental stress. This stops when pressure or worry is overcome.

Chronic insomnia: this might last a long time. It is caused mainly by secondary insomnia, a symptom of other diseases.

There are numerous reasons for insomnia. Depression and other psychological factors are the most common causes. Individuals with a significant amount of life stress, depression, psychosis, etc. typically have a poor sleep. Some physical discomfort or illnesses can also be an additional factor like heart, kidney, liver, pancreas, digestive system, etc. Problems such as respiratory diseases, cardiovascular disease, chronic pain, menopause, diabetes, arthritis, etc. can disturb healthy sleep. Some people have a problem called restless leg syndrome or a periodic limb movement disorder, which gives them a shrieking sensation when keeping their limbs idle, forcing them to move their arms involuntarily even during sleep. There can be issues such as psycho-physiological factors that stress about not sleeping. This can also lead to sleeplessness.

Certain environmental factors, such as light, sound, temperature, humidity, stale air, etc., may disturb your sleep. Lifestyle and behavior can also be a source of sleeplessness. Sedentary activity, daytime sleep, irregular sleep, and drug use, alcohol, caffeine, etc., can reduce your sleep as well. Many medicines such as over-the-counter medications or prescription drugs for fever, asthma, anxiety, allergies, high blood pressure, etc. can lead to sleeplessness. The circadian rhythm disorder caused mainly by jet delays and night shift problems is another problem. Traveling through various time zones in the aircraft could disturb the organic clock of the body and give you nights without sleep. Night shifts can cause problems until you have this routine changed.

If you have insomnia, you may have several signs and symptoms. Most of the time, you will find it difficult to fall asleep. You can wake up while sleeping and then find it hard to sleep. Some may wake up early in the morning, while others may feel sleepy during the day. Upon waking, you can feel general tiredness and decreased motor coordination. If you have insomnia, you can have fatigue, irritability, concentration problems, and poor memory.

You have to try to follow a few habits from your side before going to the sleeping pills that are not so good for your health. Keep a regular time to go to bed and wake. Don't go to sleep at the time of the day. Always do workouts, but never before you go to bed because exercise can cause you not to sleep. Take light foods before you go to sleep. Stay comfortable with your bedroom, and make it quiet, silent, and dry. Try reading books and listening to light music before bed, which can worsen your somnolence. You wake up all night with alcohol, nicotine, caffeine, etc. before bed, so stop it.

The above exercises will typically solve acute insomnia. If you feel tired and sleepy during the day, it is a problem for you. A doctor may prescribe some medications that are not very strong for a few days. In this scenario, never go for over-the-counter medicines that can have adverse side effects and also lose their effectiveness during continuous use. In the case of chronic insomnia, you must consult the doctor to determine the root cause of the problem and take the appropriate measures to cure it. The underlying cause can be demonstrated by behavioral therapies, lifestyle changes, and medical treatment. If you use any drug, don't forget to tell your doctor because it can be causing insomnia.

Let us address those drugs used for treating insomnia now. Benzodiazepine sedatives such as Halcion, Restoril, ProSom, Dalmane and Ativan, and non-benzodiazepine sedatives such as Ambien, Lunesta, and Sonata are some of the sleep drugs available nowadays. Although they give you enough sleep, they have side effects and are also addictive. The significant components of over-the-counter medicines are antihistamines. We have the effect of sleepiness and dry mouth at night. There are also antidepressant drugs available for people with depression today. All of these medications can cause various side effects, such as poor coordination, stomach problems, poor memory, problems with vision, nausea, etc. The best way to do this is to take natural treatments.

Several of the natural substances, such as 5-hydroxytryptophans, choline bitartrates, phosphatidylcholine, S-adenosyl-methionine, D-phenylalanine, hops, valerian extract, chamomile, passion flora, etc. are found to provide relaxation and sleep.

CHAPTER EIGHT

The Benefits of Sleep During Pregnancy

Only a woman can do one thing, and that has a baby. I don't think anybody's going to argue with us! And it's the most incredible thing for women. It's an exciting time, but a new life can also be very tiring. Your wellbeing needs to ensure you get plenty of sleep during pregnancy.

Several things occur during pregnancy when it comes to health. One of the first things the doctor can do when you're pregnant is to begin taking prenatal supplements to get the extra vitamins and nutrients the body needs to support a fetus. Most of the vitamins your body receives from your diet are used for your baby. This is why prenatal vitamins must be taken for optimal health during pregnancy.

The amount of sleep you get while you are pregnant will significantly affect your working time. Studies have shown that women who sleep less than 6 hours per night during their pregnancy are employed about 29 hours when those who sleep for over 7 hours have an average working life of about 17 1/2 hours. Studies also show that women who have slept less than 5 hours per night are more likely to have a C-section.

There may be many things to disrupt your sleep in the evening, such as numerous urinary trips to the bathroom, concerns about the events of the day, and overall discomfort while you are pregnant. You must take additional measures to ensure that while you are pregnant, you get as much sleep as possible. You can help improve your health during pregnancy by following the following tips.

You should assist your body with a routine for your sleeping hours. This may take a while, but it's worth the effort. The body is accustomed to the time of the night and how much sleep you need. You will find that your body is used to your set sleep time so that you can sleep longer.

You can decide to go to bed earlier in the afternoon to get a good night's sleep. Keep to it once you make the schedule. It can help to make you comfortable using a pregnancy sleeping pillow. Most of these pillows are body pillows, placed around your body to make you as comfortable as possible.

It also works a lot when making your bedroom beautiful, dark and calm, a nice place to retire in the evening. Some women say they have tired their bodies and relieved their stress through exercises during pregnancy and have a good night's rest. Make sure your room is as cold as you need it to sleep in. Pregnant women suffer from hot flushes, and this can keep them up during the night. Your wellbeing is of utmost importance during childbirth, which is why you should try to relax fully during the night.

Pregnancy and Sleep: Ways to Get the Rest You Need

Even if you've always been a great sleeper, you can change anything. In some cases, the body trains you to feed and take care of your baby at night. In the third quarter, wakefulness and insomnia are usual. Consult these recommendations, though, to get enough rest.

1) Assess your food and drink. Smoking and alcohol use based on harm to your baby should be avoided, but another reason exists. Nicotine and alcohol can lead to less restful sleep, thereby avoiding both.

Staying hydrated is essential in your pregnancy, but you should try to take your fluids early in the morning so your bladder does not prematurely wake you up.

Try avoiding heartburn and indigestion foods, especially before bedtime. Instead of eating a large evening meal, eating smaller meals during the day can help. If you have a sick morning, eating a small protein snack before dining can help soften your morning nausea or keep crackers or biscuits on the bed before even getting out of bed. Staying hydrated is essential in your pregnancy, but you should try to take your fluids early in the morning so your bladder does not prematurely wake you up.

Try avoiding heartburn and indigestion foods, especially before bedtime. Instead of eating a large evening meal, eating smaller meals during the day can help. If you have a sick morning, eating a small protein snack before dining can help soften your morning nausea or keep crackers or biscuits on the bed before even getting out of bed.

2) Sleep If you can do it, try a midday sleep of 30-60 minutes. During your pregnancy, you will feel better and less fatigued. Schedule your naptime for an hour or less, or it can bother you when you try to sleep later at night. Sleep early in the afternoon, too, so you can have a reasonable time to bed.

3) Start your day with a workout, but ensure that you start your day with exercise. It is suitable for recovery. Too late in the day can release chemicals that keep you awake or prevent you from going into a deep sleep cycle. If possible, make sure that your training ends at least four hours before you turn in. Take your partner for a nightly walk of 15-30 minutes. You're going to sleep well.

4) Write Down Your Worries You probably toss and turn all night if you lie awake thinking about everything you're going to get ready for baby birth or let you are to-dodo list cloud your thoughts. Keep a notepad next to your bed, and if needed, take a look at a couple

of items you are disturbed or want to fix. You can remember what you have to do without disturbing your sleep.

5) Practice Relaxation Learn how to relax (deep belly breathing) and practice for 5 minutes before and after bedtime. Then concentrate on relaxing your muscles, starting through the muscles in your face.

If you are concerned that you have to deal with the next birth at night, enroll in a birth class to get your questions answered and your fears squeezed. Just knowing what to expect or what other people have experienced can make you more comfortable with work, delivery, breastfeeding, and newborn care. If you are concerned that you have to deal with the next birth at night, enroll in a birth class to get your questions answered and your fears squeezed. Just knowing what to expect or what other people have experienced can make you more comfortable with work, delivery, breastfeeding, and newborn care.

7) Create a bedtime routine. Just like you're going to do for your son, create your bedtime routine. Take a bath, read a book, stop television, or look at your mobile and keep your routine regular so your body needs it.

8) Sleep as much as you can; try to go to bed, and stand up every day at the same time. Render your room a spot that you want with comfortable bedding, low lighting, better ventilation, and no TV entertainment.

9) Stay out of bed when you don't sleep If you're watching TV in bed or surfing the Internet, consider avoiding. The bed should be

reserved for sleep and sex, so consider avoiding the bed if you don't want to do either. That way, the body will know when you lie down that it's time for bed.

10) Sleeping on your left side facilitates good circulation and distribution of nutrients and will help your body quickly get rid of waste and water. Try to get used to this position early in your pregnancy, so when your belly gets bigger, it's easier.

What if I don't get to sleep?

It is normal to have disrupted sleep and even insomnia during childbirth. If you can't fall or sleep, get up, read or listen for a while to soothing music and go back to bed once you feel sleepy again.

Why Sleep Loss Could someone get Belly Fat

Diet and loss of weight have outperformed baseball as U.S national pastime. 2/3 of all U.S citizens are estimated to be overweight, 1/3 to be obese. Apart from the regular bulges that see outwards, the appearance of belly fat, not the flabby fat that is located deep within your stomach, that is connected to your intestine, is intended to increase the risk of cardiovascular disease, obesity, metabolic syndrome, higher blood pressure, colon cancer and breast cancer in female disorders.

The press and the public have almost come to see belly fat as a cause of all these medical conditions rather than just a combination with the news about the importance of belly fat as a risk factor for cardiac diseases and other medical conditions. The real question is, what starts with belly fat?

Any stress, whether internal or physical, may cause drastic physiological changes. The connection between stress and belly fat. When you are under pressure, the sympathetic nervous system or the classic fight or flight response is triggered. Besides, this will divert blood from less essential parts of the body and structures such as your gastrointestinal system, reproductive organs, hair, and distant limbs. It is like a lion-every nerve chases you, and your being's fiber will concentrate on getting away rather than digesting what you had for lunch.

While you are not likely to be hunted by a lion, any prolonged stress that leads to low blood flows to the intestines causes biochemical changes that lead to belly fat build-up. Increased estrogen released by belly fat is believed to further suppression the levels of natural progesterone in both men and women, exacerbating even the vicious cycle. The press and the public have almost come to see belly fat as a cause of all these medical conditions rather than just a combination with the news about the importance of belly fat as a risk factor for cardiac diseases and other medical conditions. The real question is, what starts with belly fat?

Any stress, whether internal or physical, may cause drastic physiological changes. The connection between stress and belly fat. When you are under pressure, the sympathetic nervous system or the classic fight or flight response is triggered. Besides, this will divert blood from less essential parts of the body and structures such as your gastrointestinal system, reproductive organs, hair, and distant limbs. It is like a lion-every nerve chases you, and your being's fiber will concentrate on getting away rather than digesting what you had for lunch.

While you are not likely to be hunted by a lion, any prolonged stress that leads to low blood flows to the intestines causes biochemical changes that lead to belly fat build-up. Increased estrogen released by belly fat is believed to further suppression the levels of natural progesterone in both men and women, exacerbating even the vicious cycle.

Poor Circulation Can Benefit Belly Fat No severe medical condition is needed to cause these rapid changes in the flow of the intestines. Even your emotional condition and the various stresses you experience every day can affect your gut and stomach flow significantly.

Researchers found that low oxygen periods in the intestines can lead to biochemical changes leading to fat accumulation. Is this low oxygen level the product of typical cardiac atherosclerosis, or is something else possible? Does anything else cause intestinal hypoxia?

As I explain in my sleep-breathing theory, it is difficult for modern people to adequately breathe during sleep at night, mainly while sleeping behind us and when they are in a deep sleep due to muscle relaxation. This is due to a slow but significant reduction in our jaws due to a major dietary change and the addition of other nutritional supplies, such as infant bottles and pacifiers.

The smaller the jaws, the less space for the tongue, and the more likely it is during deep sleep, especially when it sleeps flat and in a deep sleep. In the evening, we all fall in this spectrum, depending on how often the tongue collapse obstructs our breathing, and the severe end is legally referred to as obstructive sleep apnea. It is not surprising that irregular breathing periods, whether very short or 10 to 30 seconds (apneas), are known to cause stress.

And this constant pressure will slow down our metabolic rates, making it harder to lose weight if it doesn't gain weight.

Hormones and weight gain There is another major factor in women, which can increase the weight as you grow older. This is the function of progesterone decrease, which starts at the end of the thirties and the start of thirties.

Progesterone is an effective stimulant of the upper airway muscles, which mostly relax or strengthen the tongue, especially in a deep sleep. This is why, when progesterone levels decline during the perimenopausal period, women do not sleep as before menopause. A relative change in the sleeping condition of a woman then can result in neurological symptoms, such as night sweats, hot blows, gaining weight, mood swings, and irritability. Not very unexpectedly, even young men who move up the sleep respiration scale may experience the same symptoms. Deep or sufficient sleep is a significant cause of physiological stress.

There are seven women who were overweight and asked them to do something for four weeks: sleep more. Sleep Your Way to Weight Loss They all lose 7 to 21 pounds without making any other adjustments. Sleeping longer is one of the ways of restoring health to our deprived culture of sleep, but increasing sleep efficiency during sleep is another way of increasing your energy, improving your health, and losing weight.

Not only your breathing problem can't get well when you sleep at night and don't sleep long enough, but many other factors also stop you from having a quality sleep you need; eating late close to bedtime is a regular, modern routine for a variety of reasons. Gastric juices still lingering from your final meal (or snack) may be sucked into the throat, causing swelling, inflammation, and blockages. Alcohol in the bedtime induces more inflammation of your throat muscles, which leads to more frequent discomfort and anticipation, and more profound and prolonged snoring.

The best way to lose weight Before you start a new diet or use your new gym, make sure you can breathe in the evening. If your nose is stuffy for any excuse, do everything you can to straighten it first. If for years or decades, you have had a stuffy nose, you may not know that your nasal breathing has been impaired. Proper sleep and reducing stress levels are necessary if excess belly fat is to be removed.

CHAPTER NINE

A Dieting Nightmare: Eating Before Bedtime

Dieting seems to have overtaken our national passport baseball. There are many suggested reasons for the current obesity epidemic, such as poor diet, lack of exercise, and just too much eating. But you can also determine how quickly you can lose weight or even gain weight. Your weight can as well determine how well you are breathing and sleeping. Therefore, all three of these combined factors can create a fatal cycle of weight gain, loss of sleep, and inability to respire.

Recent studies have revealed that sleep deficiency (or poor quality sleep) is linked to obesity. The less you sleep, the more typical body signals, like cortisol and leptin, change your body's appetite.

Leptin provides energy status information to brain regulatory centers. Night levels increase partly due to daily meal intake. However, leptin levels seem to decrease significantly at night in sleep-deprived persons. The hormone which stimulates the consumption of hunger and food, or cortisol, on the other hand, has been found to increase in response to experimental sleep deprivation and insomniacs.

It is known that lower leptin levels, the hormone that tells the body when enough cortisol is consumed (especially by night). Therefore, when the leptin level decreases, as in sleeping people, it causes the cortisol level to increase, making you eat more. Besides, when you don't sleep well, Ghrelin, another hormone that makes you want to eat, goes up too. Sleep deprivation has been shown to affect the thyroid-stimulating hormone or TSH significantly. Because thyroid levels affect your metabolism, this also affects your weight.

Sleep loss has also been found to increase blood sugar levels. Add to this the high cortisol level, which is also known to increase the sugar level. As you can see, your sleep loss can cause a whole host of hormonal fluctuations, which can slow your dietary efforts. But the consequences of what I have just described are only the tip of the iceberg. If you also don't breathe well while you are sleeping, you may lose weight.

When you try to lose weight, you must be able to breathe well during the night while you are sleeping. Although many of us consider this, many patients who are thin and not overweight nevertheless find that they are rapidly gaining weight, without a substantial increase in caloric intake, if they are previously prone to a narrow airway and have difficulty breathing during sleep. Many of my patients who suffer from the sleep condition UARS (Upper Airway Resistance Syndrome), therefore, compensate by sleeping sideways or stomachs and remaining active because these are preventive measures.

But over the years, something happens to trigger a slow slope descent that makes the weight gain slightly worse. Even a couple of pounds for these patients could make a big difference, because slight weight gain in the throat reduces the fat cells in the throat, causing the soft tissue in the throat to grow inside and interfere on the airways. This exacerbates more palate or language collapse causing more excitement or apnea. This, in turn, causes sleep inefficiency, which spins out the whole metabolism that I have previously described. Moreover, you start to have more apneas as you get more weight, which can lead to other health problems such as high blood pressure.

Why can't I sleep? Why can't I?

Sleep is the first thing sacrificed in this fast-paced, stressful society when we are short on time. It is estimated that people in America sleep about 1 and 1/2 to 2 hours less per night compared to 50 years ago. Although it seems to be a small amount, any sleep shortage can accumulate in something called the "sleep debt," which is increasingly difficult to repay over time. I am not surprised to add to the poor dietary habits and the vicious cycle I described an earlier and less physical activity that far more than 50% of adults in this country are considered obese.

Diets: What am I going to lose?

It is, therefore, understandable why so many dietary programs are sold in this country. From diet pills to regiments for practice, there are a wide variety of choices to help you lose weight. What is better to note, however, is that you don't want to keep weight off once you lose it (most likely, because your products are useless as soon as you lose weight). There's undoubtedly none I know you need to breathe and sleep well to keep your ideal weight. They assume that if you are "medically qualified," your weight-loss regiment is subject to these and other health factors. But as I continuously stress patients, it will be difficult to maintain weight loss if you have a sleep breathing problem, which is not addressed too.

Therefore, my general recommendation in terms of diet is to avoid anything that stresses one thing or reduces it too much. On the contrary, eat a variety of whole foods (natural, unprocessed foods without chemicals, preservatives, or additives as close as possible to the source). It's not what you eat (or don't), but the most important thing is what you eat at what time and how often.

Consider your typical Sumo wrestler's diet, for example. Sumo wrestlers eat only one large meal a day. They also skip breakfast, which reduces their metabolism and practices intensely throughout the day. After hungering all day, they consume large amounts of food (typically high in calories) just before they go to bed. This causes enormous stress on their bodies, as you can imagine, which reacts in turn by going into "hunger mode," which mainly promotes the long-term storage and production of fat. You don't want to happen something if you try to lose weight. However, after hearing this from many patients over and over, I know that this kind of "diet" is too common for many of you.

Eating before bedtime Just before bedtime is probably the most common habit, I can see that the sleep-breathing weight gain cycle can exacerbate. Think of it like this. The narrower your airway is, the more prone it is to collapse. You take a couple of breaths into your throat if your tongue occasionally falls and you obstruct, (more likely on your back), causing an enormous vacuum effect that pulls the stomach content into your throat. If more acid is present because you only eat a meal, then you get more acid to suck into your throat, which then irritates your throat and causes more swollenness, which makes you breathe less efficiently that causes you to sleep less. This vicious cycle continues to make your loss of weight very difficult.

Most dietitian experts recommend eating a large number of small meals evenly spread (4-5 meals), rich in low glycemic food. The glycemic index is a measure of the swift absorption of sugar into the bloodstream. Foods like pasta and white rice can be quickly processed and absorbed into the bloodstream, while the glycemic indexes of barley and soy milk take a longer time to digest and to release the sugar to the blood. With low glycemic foods, just after you eat, you won't feel hungry.

So why are so many people who have a diet and exercise so difficult to lose weight? I'm willing to bet that they don't sleep long enough, or something prevents them from getting deep sleep, such as a problem for sleep respiration, if you look closely at their sleeping habits. Anecdotally, several patients with sleep-related breathing disorders and overweight experience a weight loss as soon as they are treated for sleep. So, make sure you have a good sleep hygiene program the next time you start your diet program. This could make the difference between weight loss or weight loss and keeping it safe.

Yourself Evening Hypnosis – Better Night Sleep

How does one help with sleeping hypnosis? We live in an ever more chaotic world; our jobs require more of us; our families demand more of us; we are flooded with life. It is when the lights go out we have to sleep before the next day.

But we're laying there and can't sleep no matter how hard we try, it's awful. Why? Why? Due to the lack of sleep, the mind is still working on all the stress and concerns of the day.

Sleeping hypnosis could benefit here; it speaks to the unconscious mind directly. In a session, you are advised to relax, use scripts and imagination, and transfer the conscious mind into the deeper unconscious. You can change your behavior in a hypnotic state to do something different.

Millions of people have used hypnosis to develop their confidence, overcome anxiety and phobia, stop smoking, and lose weight and can now be used to help people with insomnia. You can also take what you have learned in a session and start with self-hypnosis in the privacy of your home if you understand the process of sleeping hypnosis.

Prepare your bed, get comfortable, and shut your eyes regularly. The first thing to do is to relax. Don't worry if you don't get it the first time, and only more stress is caused by worry. Remember, this worked for many people, and it's the same for you. You will soon feel better than ever before. Be careful and gentle with yourself.

You are ready for the next step once you're in a light hypnotic state between sleep and awake, suggestions, either in the form of the session CD or the scripts created for yourself.

Scripts are the lines that you build that speak about what you want for yourself. Make them progressive and current, focus only on what you want, not what you don't want.

Don't say,' I don't want sleepless nights,' for example.

Say then,' I'm very relaxed and very well asleep.'

When it sounds too lofty, you can be idealistic, this is your particular time with your unconscious mind. In the end, it will help you out. It's also all right if you fall asleep; that's your goal.

Sleeping hypnosis is non-addictive so that you can stop the disease whenever you want and can influence your health in the future too.

You don't have to deal again with insomnia. Through taking a sleep hypnosis technique and adapting it to your private self-hypnosis, you can still enjoy a good night's sleep, which helps you to focus on your subconscious mind using scripts. By understanding the effect of these hypnotic suggestions on your mind and behavior, one really can relax and wake up to feel fresh and focused the next day.

Hypnosis is used to stop smoking, weight loss, conquer of phobia and fears, create confidence, etc. So how is hypnosis sleeping different?

Life always becomes busy as time passes; bills have to be paid, and families are taken care of. We must always be on the move, but after a long day, we must relax and recharge our batteries.

We lie for ages, however, but nothing happens. We know we have to be up in about five hours, but we can't sleep for some reason, and as we stress about it more and think about it more, things get worse. How we're going to feel tomorrow is an awful thought.

The reason this happens is that we are still in a depressed emotional state of mind, which we have been throughout the day.

In a sleeping hypnosis session, we learn how to calm the conscious mind and use suggestions to communicate directly with the unconscious. By teaching the mind to relax and we can sleep deeply, except for the tips.

If at first, you find it hard to relax, keep in mind that any new thing takes time and patience, but you will succeed. It's worked for millions, and yes, it will work for you as well. Go with comfort, and don't worry.

Only lie on your pillow, shut your eyes, and concentrate on your breath, begin a gentle 10-1 countdown on each exhalation. You'll be in a hypnotic condition; it's like being between sleep and waking.

The next thing is the suggestions submitted. If you have a qualified sleeping hypnotic session, to begin with, you may be able to obtain a CD recording that you can start at home. You could write your own, on the other hand.

Try to speak today, to advance in straightforward language. Only focus on what you want, not what you don't want. You might say,' I'm very relaxed and sleeping sound,' instead,' I don't want sleepless nights anymore.'

Believe it works, you're going to end up just as your thoughts dictate and soon feel better. Also, if you doze off when it's fine under hypnosis, the job is done.

This is your sleeping hypnosis, so it's non-addictive and, like all treatments which deal with mental wellbeing, in the years to come, it will give you extra value.

We all have to unwind after a stressful day and recharge the batteries. Sleep is a natural part of life, and something needs to be done if we have issues with it.

With self-hypnosis, we could unwind and squeeze into our subconscious and allow us to sleep and be fresh the next day. Imagine never again having insomnia? The only real answer is sleeping hypnosis.

CONCLUSION

It is not difficult to hypnotize someone immediately, but your success needs to be confident in yourself. In a few easy steps, hypnosis can be applied to anyone. Next, ensure that your environment is conducive to your subject being hypnotized. This means dimming the lights and making sure that there are no distractions, perhaps lighting some fragrant candles. Get your subject comfortable by gradually breathing into your nose and expanding out of your mouth.

Then they get rid of all emotions, worries, or doubts by assigning each of them a color, and then eject them as they breathe in and out. Now ask the person to imagine a liquid that fills them from the feet to the head, and they will feel relaxed and comfortable when this happens. An idea, a thought, or even an action can now be suggested. This is known as the hypnotic proposal. Visualization usually involves recognizing the wrong aspects of custom and then positive results when your custom is being dumped and when your subject feels far better. After the person is allowed to stay in this "happy place," it's time to return. Hypnosis is helpful for people with sleep disorders, especially sleep hypnosis.

Sleep hypnosis may lead to managing a variety of sleep disturbances. Some sleep disorders respond well to sleep hypnosis, such as bed weather, sleep insomnia, or sleepwalk.

Bed wetting affects people of all ages. Sleep hypnosis may lead to the identification and resolution of the issue. Sleeplessness also reacts well. This sleep disorder can be caused by psychological disturbances, anxiety, or medication. Therapists can relieve stress and calm fear in nightmares, which is the cause of these awful dreams.

Sleepwalking, also recognized as sleepwalking, takes place at any age. It usually happens during deep sleep for the human. While self-hypnosis may help an individual with minor sleep deprivation, a professional should better diagnose and treat short-term and long-term disorders. Sleep hypnosis fits with other therapies, such as counseling, medications, or a sleep diary.